D0817796

Lies & Myths About Corporate Wellness

BY GREG JUSTICE, MA

Copyright © 2013 GREG JUSTICE

All rights reserved. No part of this publication may be reproduced, stored in a retrieval system, or transmitted in any form or by any means, electronic, photocopying, recording, or otherwise without prior written permission, except in the case of brief excerpts in critical reviews and articles. For permission requests, contact the author at gregjustice@aycfit.com or write to:

Greg Justice
7830 State Line Road #101
Prairie Village, KS 66208

All rights reserved.
ISBN: 147018138X
ISBN-13: 978-1470181383
The author disclaims responsibility for adverse effects or consequences from the misapplication or injudicious use of the information contained in this book. Mention of resources and associations does not imply an endorsement.

Cover design: Doug Coonrod

For Dana,
David, Kale, Mia,
and Jeff

ACKNOWLEDGMENTS

During the past three decades, I've been blessed to work in the corporate wellness, health, and fitness industry. I've spent time with some of the top CEO's in the world and have learned so much about what makes them successful. One common theme is their willingness to take chances when many others won't.

I remember the advice I was given by one CEO early in my career. When so many others told me to play it safe and find a 9 to 5 job, he said "Why play it safe, if you have a dream? You're at such a great age to fail, because you've got so much time to learn, grow, and succeed." His words resonated with me and continue to challenge me to take chances, while others "play it safe."

Thank you to all the mentors who have encouraged me along the way, including Richard Rostenberg, Tim Schliebe, Dave Seitter, Harold Tivol, Julia Kauffman, John Mueller, and Tom & Jeanne Olofson. Your support and encouragement have provided a foundation of strength that serves me well today.

Thank you to my wife, Dana, whose support, friendship, and love has propelled me every step of our journey together. I love you!

Thanks to Doug Coonrod for his graphic design and to Nancy McDonald for proof-reading, editing, and publishing.

I also want to thank the wonderful AYC associates who have served our corporate clients with such professionalism throughout the years; Glen Haney, Nadine Price-Rojas, Derek Newman, Ellen Breeding, and Sean Dill.

And, finally, to the corporations that "get it." It is because of their understanding that a healthy workforce equals a more productive workforce that allows us to do what we do.

CONTENTS

INTRODUCTION

As you know, your most valuable asset is your work force. To get the most out of your business, you MUST get the most productivity out of your people.

In a nutshell, the healthier your employees are, the more and better work they can do for you, and the better their quality of life will be. Happy employees create healthy companies.

The recognition of this truism has led to a business practice generally known as "corporate wellness." But, the world of corporate wellness is rife with common myths, misperceptions, and outright lies regarding programs that encourage and promote wellness. So much so that many companies are hesitant to put a program in place.

This book will dispel the myths and lies, teach you to separate fact from fiction, and most importantly, provide you with critical guidelines for developing and managing your own successful corporate wellness program so you can maximize your investment in the human resources that make or break your business.

Lies & Myths About Corporate Wellness

1. Healthcare costs are going up, and there is nothing we can do about it.

2. What my employees do on their own time is none of my business.

3. People get sick. It's out of their control.

4. A wellness program is too expensive.

5. It takes too much time.

6. Corporate wellness is a touchy-feely new age thing that doesn't really have any solid benefit.

7. We don't have the facilities for exercise.

8. My employees won't want to do it.

9. It's too hard to know if a program is working.

I'm sure you've heard at least a few of these statements from business colleagues. But what's the real truth of the matter?

Let's tackle these statements one at a time.

Healthcare costs are going up, and there's nothing we can do about it.

Healthcare costs are rising, but a sound corporate wellness program gives you an opportunity to minimize the effects on your business. There are many factors that contribute to the increase of healthcare costs, and related health insurance costs. Many of them are beyond your control. But what is within your control is utilization (the frequency and level expenses associated with use of healthcare insurance benefits). The healthier your group is the better insurance rates you will enjoy. This also applies to your workers' compensation costs. The fewer injuries your staff incurs, the less expensive your workers' compensation insurance will be. Savings from workers' compensation and health insurance costs for healthy workers can range from 10% to 30% compared to others in your industry who have less healthy employees.

1. What my employees do on their own time is none of my business.

Although this may sound like an appropriate separation of personal and professional life, think about the benefits to the individual and your business. If your employee comes in reeking of alcohol in the morning after a night of partying – is that none of your business? Even if he or she is not actually drunk, you might have concerns about his or her ability to function, as well as concerns about his or her influence on other staff. Sending the employee home for the day (generally without pay) is not an uncommon response to this behavior. Repeat the activity two or three times in a month, and you may suspect that the employee has a substance abuse problem. Is it your "business" yet? What an employee does on personal time does impact behavior in the workplace. An employee's lifestyle definitely impacts insurance, benefits, workers' compensation costs, and productivity. The reality is that employers historically do not view wellness and lifestyle behavior as impacting profits and productivity. This book will change that.

2. People get sick. It's out of their control.

Many illnesses are a result of lifestyle choices. Diseases such as cancer, stroke, heart disease, lung disease, and diabetes do not always occur wholly by way of bad luck. They can often develop due to chronic neglect or abuse of the body. Note that the six of the top seven causes of death in the U.S. are lifestyle diseases. The one exception is automobile accidents. A person's wellness, from the common cold to more serious diseases, or repetitive stress injuries, are usually just a result of lifestyle choices.

3. It's too expensive. My company's too small to afford a wellness program.

Wellness programs can be surprisingly inexpensive and cost-effective. The returns in reduced costs are the tip of the iceberg. Healthy employees increase productivity, focus, and energy, and having a wellness program in place creates loyalty and camaraderie from a workforce that appreciates the employer's concern and support. This leads to reduced turnover, which is yet another cost savings. An employer with just a handful of employees will benefit from these advantages.

4. It takes too much time.

Management involvement is a must for a wellness program to be successful. However, this does not need to be a time-consuming endeavor. Vendors are available to take care of all program details from setting up and running a program, to measuring the results. As for employee time commitment, much of what employees can do to participate is done outside of working hours. If you're inclined to allow extra time in the work day for your employees to exercise, so much the better. But if you cannot spare the time during the work day, they can exercise during lunch or after work with quick, effective 30-minute workout regimens.

5. It's a touchy-feely new age thing that doesn't really have any solid benefit.

Wellness programs have been studied for more than 20 years now. Their benefits are irrefutable when they are properly implemented and when the management team is committed to their success.

6. We don't have the facilities for exercise.

You don't need a gym in order to have room to exercise. You don't need thousands of dollars of complex gym equipment for your employees to exercise. Workouts can be conducted in small areas with bodyweight for resistance and be amazingly effective.

7. My employees won't participate.

Some employees won't. Many, however, are already interested in being more fit, and others will benefit from a bit of education on the matter and are quite willing to participate in a program that's easy to understand, convenient, and encouraged by their employer. Add the incentive of a reduced health insurance premium, and any other incentives you want to use to sweeten the pot, and you'll have more participation than you would have imagined.

9.   It's too hard to know if it's working

When you set up your wellness program, you can (and should) also determine what you want to achieve. Productivity metrics, healthcare cost reduction, and reduced on-the-job injuries will provide statistical evidence of the program's effectiveness over time.

Throughout this book, you will learn the why's and how-to's of effective wellness programs, and I'll explode the myths and correct the misconceptions. You'll come to understand the importance of being committed to your employees' wellness, and how to go about making sure your efforts pay off.

PART ONE

THE PROBLEM

1

THE IMPORTANCE OF WELLNESS

American employers lose more than 300 billion dollars of productivity annually due to illness, sick days, absenteeism and sub-par performance ("presenteeism").

How much did YOU lose last year?

For every dollar an employer spends on salaries and wages, they spend a minimum of an additional 10 cents on health insurance and workers compensation costs. This is above and beyond the unintentional and often unrecognized costs noted above.

Why is wellness important in the corporate environment? Why should employers be concerned about their employees' wellness?

The average employee misses 8.4 days annually due to illness or injury, totaling more than $63 billion nationwide. The employee with a serious or chronic condition (diabetes, lung disease, heart disease, cancer, etc.) misses 72 days annually, and works at diminished capacity when present. Nationwide, more than 2.5 billion work days are reduced or lost completely.

Is this the kind of workforce you intended to employ?

Have you budgeted for this reduction in productivity?

So you have employees who get sick. Everyone gets sick from time to time, right?

Maybe so, maybe no.

Even the common cold is subject to a person's immune system letting it occur, so if you have employees in stellar health, they may well not miss a single day or even be under the weather for years at a time. Which would you rather have? A workforce of vital, energetic hard-working individuals focused on results and available to work when and where you need them? Or, would you rather have a workforce of average individuals who use up most of their sick leave, (if not more than their fair share), and come to work dragging their heads and underperforming?

Wellness in the workplace has many benefits, and employers who have tracked their employees' wellness, as well as those who have contributed to their employees' wellness, have enjoyed increases in productivity, decreased healthcare costs, decreased workers compensation costs, and increased employee loyalty and higher morale.

Benefits of Wellness in the Workplace

Although good health and vitality benefit the employee in every aspect of his or her life, they also specifically benefit the employer as well. Just as investing in your employees' training provides you with a better, more valuable resource, investing in their health will provide you with a more effective and consistently available resource.

The costs associated with unhealthy employees are staggering.

"Soft costs" such as absenteeism and reduced productivity are calculated as costing four to seven times the amount that employers pay in health insurance premiums and workers compensation premiums combined. If you're a large enough employer that you self-insure these exposures, your soft costs could be an even greater multiple (based on the theory that your direct costs are less than your commercial insurance premium would be).

The American population is, sadly unhealthy. So, if your employees seem average to you, in terms of their health, they are most likely overweight, and 30% of them are obese. Many are at risk for, or already have, diabetes, high blood pressure, respiratory compromise, and/or heart disease.

Take a look at your staff. Who is overweight? Who has a flushed face and is breathing hard just walking in from the parking lot? Who are the couch potatoes? Who's on medication for high blood pressure or other chronic impairments? Bear in mind that discriminating against employees due to medical disability is certainly not encouraged and in most cases is illegal. But, we're just talking about getting a sense of the overall health of your entire staff.

If you look at your workforce from this perspective, are you pleased with what you see?

Or, do you have a rising sense of discomfort when you write out the check for your health insurance payment or your workers compensation premiums?

Or when one of your employees calls in sick for the 15th time this year with a migraine?

Rather than feel helpless, observe that perhaps migraines are a sign of stress, rather than a debilitating illness that occurs in a vacuum. Would providing stress management and exercise opportunities, and even strongly encouraging them through incentives, get you a more consistently available and performing employee?

What Is Wellness, Really?

The Random House Dictionary definition of wellness is:

1. the quality or state of being healthy in body and mind, esp. as the result of deliberate effort.

2. an approach to healthcare that emphasizes preventing illness and prolonging life, as opposed to emphasizing treating diseases.

We'll be incorporating both of those definitions into the topics discussed in this book.

Some people look at wellness simply as the absence of any apparent or disabling illness. But, being "healthy" is not simply a matter of being average in terms of having illnesses that are common and treated with over the counter drugs or with barely a raised eyebrow from the medical community.

If you look at the life insurance weight tables, you'll see numbers that reflect the average of what people actually weigh, which is **not the same as recommended healthy weights.** The casual observer believes that if his or her weight falls within those on the table, he or she must be "okay." **That is not the case.** It just means that he or she is within the statistical norm. The same disconnect exists in our perception of the health of those around us (and ourselves!). We become used to what's the norm, not what's actually healthy, and we use "normal" as the benchmark for "healthy." Unfortunately, it is not.

Vitality, energy, stamina, and systemic strength are what's healthy. Chronic disease, even low-level, missed work, repeated colds, sore throats, sinus infections, headaches, etc. are all signs of an unhealthy body. Many, if not all, of these ailments respond to wellness intervention if the employee is willing to make necessary changes.

An example of a common disease is gastroesophageal reflux disorder (GERD), and its precursor or oftentimes only noticeable symptom, heartburn. Thousands upon thousands of people suffer from this affliction. Very strong and effective medications are available to treat its symptoms, both over the counter and by prescription. It's such a frequent affliction that people don't take it very seriously.

However, notwithstanding the potentially catastrophic

medical results of chronic GERD (esophageal lesions or cancer, for example), people with GERD are found to suffer decreased productivity so severely that a recent study by the International Foundation for Functional Gastrointestinal Disorders has calculated that more than $2 billion is lost in productivity each week due to the disease. That's right – each week!

What does this have to do with wellness?

Very conveniently, two common ways to reduce or eliminate GERD are weight loss and stress reduction. Both can easily be accomplished through a good exercise regimen. A wellness program can efficiently and effectively reduce the incidence of GERD for individuals and for entire workforces. An estimated 5 - 7% of people are chronic GERD sufferers. Do you think you have any in your workforce? If you know who they are, are they overweight? High-strung? Chronic worriers? Can you see the benefit of a bit of wellness-oriented intervention?

You may think that other illnesses, such as heart disease, diabetes, cancer, and stroke are simply bad luck, and it's a shame when they happen to someone, but they cannot be prevented.

Wrong.

Living a fit and healthy life can radically minimize the incidence of such diseases. Of the top seven causes of death, six are what are called "lifestyle diseases." This means that they are caused by a person's lifestyle choices, at least in part, if not in whole.

Top 7 Causes Of Death:

Disease	Percentage of Deaths
Heart Disease	28.5%
Cancer	22.8%
Stroke	6.7%
Respiratory disease	5.1%
Accidents	4.4%
Diabetes	3%
Flu and pneumonia	2.7%

Even though we say that "accidents" are the exception to the lifestyle disease mortality percentages, even some of the accidental deaths could be prevented by wearing seat belts, not driving while impaired, or taking other precautions.

If you look at the above table and evaluate your workforce, you will no doubt find a significant percentage of employees who either suffer from or are at risk for one or more of these diseases. And while they may not succumb to disease while in your employ, chances are that their work will be negatively impacted by struggles with illness.

From a humanitarian viewpoint, you would want the best for your employees, and you would want to see them free of these dread diseases. However, there is also the very practical matter of your business's bottom line that gives you a vital interest in your employees being free of disease.

Between the time they spend at the doctor's office, the time they spend out sick, and the time they are working at less than full speed, you are losing an average of $2,000 to $2,800 per employee per year due to illnesses. These numbers don't include the healthcare costs or workers' compensation costs incurred due to illness.

Review the above table carefully, and contemplate the nature of these diseases. Think about the usual doctor's recommendations to lose weight, reduce stress, quit smoking, etc., and you will note that many of these illnesses can be mitigated or prevented entirely by a healthy lifestyle. A healthy lifestyle can be roughly defined as maintaining an optimal weight, eating right, not smoking, engaging in (at least) moderate exercise, and managing stress.

Even when it comes to such minor illnesses as the flu, a person's immune system plays a tremendous part in whether or not an illness will take hold. A healthy immune system can be developed and maintained by living a healthy lifestyle.

The relationship between a healthy diet and cardiovascular health and diabetes is even more clear, subject to the rare exceptions when a person is afflicted with a genetic or structural flaw in his or her system. Even then, taking measures to live a healthy lifestyle may prolong life and vitality.

2

DEVELOPING TRENDS
IN THE WELLNESS WORLD

If you go online and enter the search term "corporate wellness," you'll be inundated with links and advertisements from hundreds, if not thousands of wellness program vendors, and even more articles. Most of those articles tout the success and necessity of such programs. Although some articles attempt to debunk the usefulness of the programs, you will find that they tend to be written by healthcare professionals whose business will be drastically reduced if their patients become healthy.

From Dubai to Dublin to Denver, implementation of corporate wellness programs is in vogue. Much of the growth in these programs has been in the last 10 years. Wellness programs began to take hold in the 1980's, but they have taken a long time to catch on.

Part of the challenge is the recognition by healthcare insurers of the benefits of wellness programs. "Will the employees really use them? Will their health improve?" Another challenge is the regulatory issues caused by the Health Insurance Portability and Accountability Act (HIPAA) and other healthcare-related legislation that makes discounting premium for employees based on their health factors a possibly discriminatory act.

Yes, we know – not being able to discriminate based on

health factors when pricing health insurance seems a bit counterintuitive, but it's the way the laws are written now. Healthcare insurers eventually found the rationales they needed to get around those prohibitions, and interestingly, they can now provide discounts for employees who participate in certain activities without actually checking for results in the employees' health profiles. For example, a healthcare insurer may provide a credit for employees who don't smoke without regard to the actual state of their pulmonary or cardiovascular health.

One of the most common attributes for wellness programs is the Health Risk Assessment (HRA). Some programs consist of nothing more than an HRA, but for most, it is a tool for an employee to self-identify risk factors that need tending to. Some of them are apparent without any help from the HRA. For example, if an employee smokes, there's a very good chance that he or she knows it's probably not a good thing.

However, many employees are unaware of how very high-risk their status is if they smoke and have a history of stroke or heart disease in their near family, and are also overweight. An HRA can help an employee see clearly what impact his lifestyle is having on his health.

With the growth of the Internet, and the widespread acceptance by health insurers to engage in some form of wellness support, these HRAs can be taken in the privacy of the employee's home, and the results are strictly confidential. Some insurer or wellness program systems are sophisticated enough to provide recommendations for improving health based on the employee's input.

Across the board, employers who have invested in wellness programs have seen returns from 300% to 1000% on their invested dollars. These results occur not only in reduced healthcare and workers compensation costs, but reduced absenteeism and increased productivity.

This is all well and good, but what is a "wellness program?" We'll explore that thoroughly in this book. There is a surprisingly broad range of activities and services offered by wellness programs. So much so, that the choices can be overwhelming.

The good news is that this means you can structure a program to suit your needs, and which you are most likely to implement and support. The challenge is that if the program is insufficiently robust to produce favorable results, your perception of wellness programs may be forever tainted.

According to a recent MetLife survey, more than 57% of large employers (500 or more employees) and 16% of small employers offer some form of wellness program. These programs generally include smoking cessation and weight loss assistance, and 80% of these employers also provide financial incentives such as reduction in the employee's contribution to healthcare insurance, or membership at a gym.

Many small employers feel they cannot afford to engage in a wellness program. They may need to rely upon their healthcare insurer to provide most, if not all benefits.

Employee Participation

A 2008 study by Maritz, an employee motivation consultant, indicates that 16% of employees participate at least once a week in a wellness program activity, given no incentive to do so. If an incentive is provided for obtaining certain goals, that number jumps up to 23%. The study also shows that these participating employees are more loyal to and engaged with their employer, and they miss significantly less work than their non-participating co-workers.

The Wellness Culture

One of the variables not addressed in the Maritz study was the level of wellness culture at the various employers surveyed. It would be interesting to note the participation percentages where management was fully engaged in the wellness challenge and actively encouraged participation, versus those where the wellness program is merely offered to the employee for his or her usage if desired.

Dating back to the days of the musclemen on Venice Beach, and the crazy runners of the 1970's, there has always been a small cross-section of the population that looked at their bodies and decided to be proactive in creating a stronger, healthier one. These people taking an active interest in their health have been in the minority. Today, we are seeing a polarization in the United States, where more than 70% of the population is overweight (about half of those obese) and the remaining percentage seem to be at the gym.

People who are just "naturally" in shape or healthy are mostly limited to those engaged in physical labor, and certainly no longer consists of a large portion of young people, as obesity in children has reached epidemic proportions.

Despite the glut of "healthy" drinks, food, and pill advertisements on TV and in "health" magazines, along with exercise DVD's and equipment, there is not much of a wellness culture permeating the country. However, there are pockets of wellness, as indicated by the proliferation of gyms, spas, fitness centers, and fitness classes that thrive in many demographic areas.

But, if the population does not want to become fit or stay fit on its own, what is an employer to do with his workforce?

Developing a wellness culture within your own workplace can be a daunting task. Most importantly, it must start at the top. It is challenging for employees to take the exhortations of their managers to "become healthier" seriously if the boss is an overweight smoker who cannot make it up the stairs in the morning without stopping for rest breaks. (You may want to stop here for a moment if this describes you, and contemplate moving forward with changes in your own life to help yourself, as well as your employees and your company.)

If you and your management team are committed to healthier lifestyles for yourselves, and committed to your company supporting and encouraging all employees to achieve healthier lifestyles, then you're halfway down the road to creating a wellness culture.

As a practical matter, a wellness culture within a company can manifest in many ways, some of them a bit subtle. For example, if you have vending machines at work, are they filled only with chips, cookies and soft drinks? Or, do you also offer options such as fresh fruit, rice cakes and vegetable juices? If you have a company cafeteria, are low-fat and low-salt options available for your employees? If only fast food restaurants are near your office, do you offer employees a refrigerator so they can bring their own healthy lunches? Do you allow them sufficient time to go to healthier restaurants?

If a group of employees wanted to start walking after work, would you allow them to come in a little earlier during winter months so it would still be light when they left to walk? Might you provide flexible hours for employees who exercise on their lunch hour? Or are you willing to let those who want to exercise right after work take a shorter lunch? Could you create a team of employees who participates in walk-a-thons or a softball, soccer or volleyball league?

Would you be willing to institute a reward system or contest for exercise/wellness pursuits? A reserved parking spot for the person who exercised most consistently the previous month? Or, a Biggest Loser reward for the person who lost the most weight during the year?

Many of these endeavors are inexpensive, if they cost

anything at all, and once you start thinking "how can I support all of us getting healthier?" you will be amazed at the number of options that present themselves.

You can also ask your employees what would motivate them, and what activities or reward systems they would most like to participate in. Their creativity might surprise you.

If the desire to be healthy starts from the top down, it will infiltrate all layers of management and workforce. Once it becomes the expected norm, many more employees will assume the same attitude, if for no other reason than that they want to fit in. It can be quite disconcerting to be the only person sitting at a desk eating fried chicken when everyone else is exercising and eating healthy lunches, looking and feeling better than they ever have and reaping the rewards of whatever incentive programs you may have instituted. Do not be afraid to take advantage of peer pressure in encouraging your employees to participate. Naturally, those with a disability or a medical contraindication to exercise must be treated accordingly.

Legislation Trends

Obesity and other health concerns have reached such epidemic proportions that the federal government is looking at stepping in to provide motivation, guidelines, or incentives that will encourage employers to make wellness a higher priority in the workplace.

There are two bills pending in Congress that have not yet

passed but may well become law in the near future.

The Wellness and Prevention Act of 2007 (HR 853) provides for a wellness program tax credit for employers that develop and implement a program that provides certain services. The Act even extends a tax credit to participating employees.

The Healthy Workforce Act of 2007 (S 1753) provides a tax credit for an employer offering a "qualified wellness program."

In September of 2008, the House of Representatives passed a resolution declaring the first week of April to be "National Workplace Wellness Week" in recognition of the importance of health promotion in the workplace.

Also in September of 2008, the Senate passed a resolution recognizing the importance of workplace wellness as a strategy to help maximize employees' health and well being.

For many years, employers have felt it is the employees' responsibility to care for their own wellness, to find the time to exercise, eat right, relieve stress and so on. However, many people, including some of the most unwell employees, spend more time working than they do in any other single activity, so it's easy to see why the government would feel that it is becoming the employers' responsibility to ensure that there are tools offered to the employees to facilitate better health.

Once an individual is out of school, work is the only other place the government can imagine they will consistently be. They have relied on the medical community to keep our population healthy for many years, but that isn't working very well. One can hardly blame them for looking at alternatives.

At the same time, employers must be cognizant of the privacy laws and rights surrounding health and medical conditions, and the protections against discrimination that exist for those who suffer from a disability.

The Impact of the Affordable Care Act on Corporate Wellness Programs – Good, Bad, or Unknown?

One of the major thrusts of the Patient Protection and Affordable Care Act (PPACA) is an increased focus on prevention and wellness, as opposed to a historical federal focus on responding to disease and injury as they become apparent and reach epidemic proportions. Although there are many unknowns, both in the application of the PPACA, and the effect of prevention and wellness programs on individuals making lifestyle choices, wellness programs are seen as one of the few constructs available that might modify behavior and result in a healthier population overall.

Only time will tell whether the intersection of the PPACA and the concept of employer-sponsored wellness programs net a discernible benefit or interrupts current momentum in the growth of such programs.

The Affordable Care Act certainly acknowledges the

existence and benefits of employer-based wellness programs. From 2011 to 2015 the Act provides $200 million in grant funds to assist small employers with the implementation of wellness programs. "Small employers" are defined as those with fewer than 100 employees working 25 or more hours per week. The grants are eligible only for those employers who have not already embarked upon a wellness program, and other criteria apply.

In addition to these grants, the PPACA provides for technical assistance to employers seeking to implement and manage a wellness program and will be conducting surveys and studies regarding wellness program structures and results throughout the nation.

Another provision in the Act increases the health insurance premium discounts an employer can extend to employees who participate in wellness programs. Prior to the passage of the Act, such discounts were limited to 20% of the cost. Under the Act, the discount can now be up to 30%, and may even reach 50% under some circumstances. Providing discounts to participants can be seen as a punitive measure taken against non-participants, and employers are required to adhere to guidelines that assure a non-discriminatory implementation of such incentives.

An acknowledgement of the importance of workplace wellness programs is implicit in their inclusion within the healthcare law. However, there are some provisions, which may not be interpreted as being quite so favorable.

The PPACA establishes prevention and public health outreaches that would appear to compete with employer-based programs. These outreaches are community-based and will be funded more aggressively than the workplace-related programs, starting at $500 million in 2010 and increasing to $2 billion in 2015. Employers will continue to fund wellness programs predominantly on their own, whether directly, or through their healthcare insurance premiums. These community-based programs may compete directly with employers and reduce participation in the employer-sponsored program. For the employees and their families, this is of little consequence, and more choice is generally a good thing for the consumer. The employees will choose the program that suits them the best, and will use it as they see fit. But for the employer, reduced participation in their workplace program could have a negative impact on their insurance pricing, even though the employees themselves are becoming healthier. Some insurance carriers require a certain percentage of employees participate in a wellness program in order to allow a discount in the company's healthcare insurance premium. If discounts are available to individual employees, an employee utilizing a program outside the employer may not be eligible. The employees that choose to use a community-based program may also be creating hardship for other employees by not participating in the employer-sponsored plan.

Employers may also find themselves thwarted in their attempts to provide wellness programs through their insurers. The PPACA mandates minimum percentages of premium dollars to be spent on clinical or quality services. A wellness program will likely not qualify as either, although the law does not specifically define those services at this time. Many insurers will need to extract their wellness programs from their suite of free value-added services and provide them only at a cost, or will terminate them altogether in order to comply with these mandates. Employers will then need to pay the insurance company separately for wellness program services or will need to contract with wellness program vendors. Either way, they will be incurring additional costs.

If an employer is faced with this decision regarding funding of the workplace wellness program at a juncture where the program has not yet proven its value in reduced absenteeism and increased productivity, it is quite possible the employer will not continue to provide such a program. And, unfortunately, since the employer was already engaged in a wellness program offering, it would be unable to qualify for one of the Act's grants to offset these increased costs so that it could continue with its program.

The Affordable Care Act also provides for a nationwide study of wellness programs, which could result in statistically meaningful information regarding outcomes, productivity, absenteeism, improvement in health characteristics and other metrics. Unfortunately, several of the metrics to be monitored by the administrators of the national study to produce this valuable information are beyond the scope of what is currently considered proper and respectful of employees' privacy regarding healthcare information in the work place.

Section 4303 of Title IV of the Act indicates the following metrics will be assessed:

Employees' health behaviors, health outcomes and healthcare expenditures; and in the health status of employees, absenteeism, productivity, rate of workplace injury, and medical costs incurred by employees.

In order to avoid even the appearance of impropriety, and to avoid any implication of discriminatory behavior, many employers studiously avoid knowledge of several of the above metrics. Employees' fear of being taken to task regarding such issues as health outcomes, healthcare expenditures and health-related absenteeism is a concern that works against employee acceptance of a wellness program in the first place. If the employer has a self-insured plan, human resources personnel take care to avoid employee-specific cost analysis to ensure employee privacy. If the plan is a commercial one, the human resources personnel tend to have less of an opportunity to come into contact with employee-specific information in the first place. Even with workers compensation claims, employee medical information is closely guarded, and the employer receives only those details needed to determine the duties to which the employee may be returned, and the probable time frame in which that return may occur.

Employees gain a significant level of comfort with wellness

programs when they understand that their participation is completely voluntary, that they won't be judged for good or ill based on whether they choose to participate, and no one is watching over them to ensure that their health improves due to participation.

This federal study will compromise the painstakingly developed reinforcement of employees' privacy in these regards and could well have a chilling effect on their desire to participate in their employer's program, even if they have been participating previously. The downside to this is obvious and multifaceted. The employees will lose the benefit of their participation in a wellness program, regardless of how marginal that benefit may have been. The employer will lose the benefit of that employee's participation in the program. The study will be skewed by the employees who prefer less intrusion into their healthcare specifics being underrepresented in the demographic studied. This does not bode well for a statistically sound result from the study. Concerns about the erosion of employees' privacy were voiced frequently prior to the passage of the Act. Reconciling those concerns with the required metrics and analysis seems a nearly impossible task.

By contrast, the community-based programs sponsored by the Prevent and Public Health Fund do not specify metrics to be gathered from subject individuals. The pertinent subsection of Title IV, Section 4003 indicates that the Community Preventive Services Task Force has the duty to assess, every five years, "...the health effects of interventions, including health impact assessment and population health modeling..."

Between the kinder, gentler evaluation of community-based programs, and the extraordinary disparity in funding, it's not hard to imagine that workplace wellness programs will quickly be eclipsed by their community-based counterparts.

For those employers that participate in PPACA-established state insurance exchanges, wellness programs may net no benefit related to insurance costs. The state insurance exchanges are allowed to utilize only very limited criteria in establishing their premium rates. Participation in wellness programs does not appear to be an authorized criterion at this time. The criteria could be subject to change, as the exchanges are not yet active, and many rules, regulations, procedures and details have yet to be formulated and promulgated.

Overall, the impact of the PPACA upon the implementation and continued use of workplace wellness programs appears to be a mixed bag. The Act is generally supportive of wellness programs, encouraging and supporting them in the workplace, the community, and for persons insured by individual plans. But the Act also brings unique pressures to bear upon wellness programs in the workplace by requiring intrusive metrics for federal analysis and creating and significantly funding competing programs.

3

THE DOWNSIDE OF BEING UNWELL... AND HOW A CORPORATE WELLNESS PROGRAM CAN HELP

Can your business afford a sick workforce?

The costs of ill health, both in premiums and in lost productivity are staggering. As mentioned earlier, it can cost up to $2,800 per employee per year. And from the statistics, many, many employees do have issues.

Even if you're a small employer, let's say 20 – 35 people, chances are the 50% or more of your staff is afflicted by some sort of chronic disease, illness, or challenge. Interestingly, depression is one of the most severe diseases in terms of costing employers sick time and lost productivity. You can use www.depressioncalculator.com to see what the likelihood is that your workforce is afflicted with depression, and calculate your lost costs from that illness alone.

If you're lucky enough to escape the depressed employee, look at your general workforce, and do these calculations:

Approximately 30% of people over 18 have high blood pressure. Of those, 50% don't know it, and of the 50% who do, treatment is not successfully controlling it. Diabetics who have high blood pressure is at a staggering 70%!

As of 2007, more than 35% of adult men are considered obese. Obesity is a precursor for several illnesses such as high blood pressure, diabetes, and heart disease. ("Obese" is defined as being more than 20% over one's ideal body weight.)

Approximately 9% of men and women suffer from some form of coronary disease.

Approximately 8 in 1,000 people suffer from diabetes.

Unless you have one very unfortunate person in your office who has all the obesity, high blood pressure, coronary disease and diabetes there is to go around, chances are you have multiple employees afflicted with disease or other conditions.

If you add non-life threatening illnesses, such as allergies, arthritis and asthma, your statistics start to look pretty grim:

- 20% of people have allergies

- 10% of the population has hay fever.

- 6.4% of people have asthma

- 13.6% of people have arthritis

- 28% of people have GERD

- .04% of people have some form of cancer.

So, what do you think the chances are that all of your

employees are healthy, and you don't need a wellness program? Can you count the likely number of employees suffering from some form of disease or illness and multiply that by $2,000? This is your real minimum cost of unwell employees.

The True Cost of An Unwell Workforce

If you could capture that lost productivity, how much more work could your employees do? How much less frequently would you need to add staff? How much less would you pay for health insurance premiums?

Next, compare your minimum cost of unwell employees to the average cost per employee of implementing a wellness program. The average cost for an effective wellness program is $100 to $150 per employee per year. The return on that investment is anywhere from $300 to $750.

Can you afford to continue without an effective wellness program?

The Magnified Risk with Key Employees

So far, the numbers we've talked about are averaged among all employees. The next thing for you to consider is something not studied separately, so you will have to use your own anecdotal evidence and musings to determine how important it is to you and what the probable costs are.

This issue is that of unwell key employees. Those key people may be business partners, senior managers, intrapreneurs, super-salespeople, or uber-productive staff members. Any of the people upon which your business turns, whether they be cheerleaders, innovators, leaders, or highly proficient technical people – you know who they are – are worth their weight in gold, and probably worth more than you're paying them.

If the average employee costs you $2,000 to $2,800 when they're down and out, what does it cost you for any of these superstars to be operating at less than full power?

Not only are you dealing with sub-par performance, and expectations possibly not being met for a period of time, you are also incurring opportunity cost because of the stellar performance that's lacking in the moment.

If you have a superstar who can barely hold his head up due to illness, depression, anxiety, etc., he will no doubt miss opportunities coming across his or her desk that would normally be seized upon.

Can you even begin to put a price tag on your opportunity costs?

What about your high-impact employees who carry a lot of weight primarily due to the sheer amount of work they can perform? If a normal employee being less productive costs you $2,000 a year – how much does a super-performer being under the weather cost?

What about your corporate cheerleaders? If you have more than 20 employees, you no doubt have someone who keeps everyone motivated and going forward - someone who brings sunshine into the office and lifts everyone's mood. Every employer has someone who loves the company and helps juice up the loyalty among the rest of the staff. What happens when he is down, dragging, or absent? You're losing more than just that individual's productivity. You're losing the buoyancy of your other staff members.

What about your business partner? The yin to your yang? If she is distracted by medical issues or less than optimally productive do things get a bit lopsided? Are you less effective? Is your company less productive?

Additionally, key employees, especially business partners, may be insured by a key man life insurance policy. This policy will provide the business with money to keep running while searching for a replacement, and to pay the salary of that replacement. If you want to insure a valued employee, the better health they're in, the less expensive that policy will be!

You can see that there are certain key individuals in your business whose health is probably more important to you than you ever thought. Anyone on whom you rely to be more than a cog in the wheel is someone you would want to see committed to achieving the highest possible level of health.

Can you force these people to participate in a wellness program if their health is so important to you? Legally, probably not. But, you can apply a great deal of encouragement, enticement, persuasion and motivation. And, as is usually the case, once they start to see the benefits of feeling better, looking better, losing weight, and breathing easier, they will want to continue on their own. Plus, they will be even more loyal to you for caring.

CEO in Action? Or CEO Inaction?

Businesses come in all shapes and sizes, much like the CEOs who run them.

The lifeblood of the business depends on the drive, the energy, and the action the CEO puts forth to provide the direction and growth for the business vision to prosper.

CEOs are the driving force behind our country's economy and commerce. They are the doers, the movers and shakers that make it all happen.

The most effective CEOs understand and acknowledge their own strengths and weaknesses and capitalize on them or compensate for them by hiring and delegating for effectiveness and completeness of their organizations. They are the leaders who provide the spark and the example for their employees to follow.

They rule like the head of a family who instills order and integrity into the group dynamics to grow up the family in the way that is most productive for them. This is similar to the school teacher who finds ways to instill the necessary information into students and then find ways for them to apply the concepts for desired outcomes.

Every department in a business is different, yet all action is directed to the same vision, the same outcome. The types of people, equipment and supplies, and methods used by each department is different

Most CEOs are reinvesting in equipment updates and insisting on faithfully following maintenance schedules to prolong productivity and life. They send their key employees to seminars and continuing education with the understanding that those employees will come back to their job function and take action to put that information or those skills into practice with action.

The same CEOs do not recognize that their own body is an organization of systems and processes, with each organ, system, bone, muscle, and joint having its own job to do, interdependent on the other organs, systems, bones, muscles, and joints. These systems can only function fully when provided with seven key ingredients - water, sleep, exercise, nutrition, fresh air, low stress, and sunshine - every day. If the human body does not receive these key elements it will break down into a state of disease and deterioration - 100% guaranteed.

CEOs are human, just like their employees, and have their own priorities and values. Many CEOs are not wellness minded, and do not take care of their own health because they are "busy."

There are many reasons why people put the care of their body and their health last in their list of priorities.

Oftentimes people don't take care of themselves until they have symptoms that interfere with their daily lives. Making money is one of those reasons. Losing income is one interference that spurs people to action.

The CEO that is motivated to implement a wellness program for employees because of the high costs of insurance, low productivity, and absenteeism, among other company problems, is no different than the person who has a heart attack and is told to start exercising and eating right or he will die. Suddenly everyone is paying attention.

The human body has 11 distinct systems that are interdependent of each other to sustain their job function. The supplies they need EVERY DAY to function well include restful sleep, water, exercise, nutrition, fresh air, stress reduction, and sunshine. Regular exercise and proper nutrition supply the foundation of these bodily needs.

When you compare the human body's systems to a company's....

Human Body Systems / Business Systems

Circulatory System (heart, blood, vessels) ....Customer Service
Respiratory System (nose, trachea, lungs) ....Advertising
Immune System ....Business Vision/Mission
Skeletal ....Business Structure and Culture
Integumentary (skin, hair, nails, glands)...........................Security
Urinary System (bladder, kidneys) .....Maintenance and Janitorial
Muscular System (muscles)...........................Sales and Marketing
Endocrine System (glands) ....Clerical and Administrative
Digestive System ....Equipment and Supplies

If a system in your business or your body is destined to break down for lack of care, which system would you agree to allow to work at a reduced capacity or to do without altogether?

I recently had a conversation with a client that is typical of the perspective of people everywhere. When I asked him if he took any medications, he said "no." I looked at him quizzically and he corrected himself, "Well, just my high blood pressure medicine." Too many people don't understand that medication is not a cure, nor a long term solution to chronic illness, and it isn't a 'normal' state of ageing. Medication is like a cast on a broken leg – it's there to help you while you take ACTION to get your body healthy again.

The Mayo Clinic states, "High blood pressure can quietly damage your body for years before symptoms develop." It continues to explain some of the complications high blood pressure can cause when it's not effectively controlled.

Complications include damage to your arteries, aneurysm, damage to your heart, heart failure, damage to your brain, stroke, dementia, kidney failure, and damage to your eyes. Other possible dangers include sexual dysfunction, bone loss, and sleep apnea.

Thousands of research studies have shown that regular exercise and proper nutrition are key ingredients to achieving health and wellness and that without them, the **body will deteriorate into a state of disease.** That disease is still present while a person is on medication and not exercising and/or eating nutritiously.

Mayo Clinic explains how high blood pressure and exercise are connected, "Regular physical activity makes your heart stronger. A stronger heart can pump more blood with less effort. If your heart can work less to pump, the force on your arteries decreases, lowering your blood pressure."

The human heart is a muscle. Regular exercise is needed to strengthen the heart as well as the body. If the leg muscles are weak, how can the heart muscles be strong? If your business sales are weak, how can your business growth be strong?

The bottom line is that every human being needs regular exercise and proper nutrition. Wellness programs are usually very good about providing lots of good information to the employees and the CEO about what it takes to create and maintain a healthy body, yet that is where most of them stop.

While the employee is expected to be taking proactive action all day, every day on their job, most wellness programs simply put the information forth and assume that the employees will take the necessary action.

Therein lies the key to wellness program success. Every organizational structure follows the leader – what is good for the goose is good for the gander, right? If a CEO is leading by "do as I say, not as I do," the wellness program has little to no chance of success.

The human body predictably follows the input and actions of the brain that is controlling it. The business predictably follows the input and actions of the CEO and upper management controlling it. Insisting that they eat well and then bringing in donuts for a meeting is counterproductive and sends a very clear message that the wellness program is lip service and not a part of the company culture and values.

According to the Centers for Disease Control, a sedentary body with poor nutritional habits describes 70% of the people who die of preventable illness each year in this country.

CEOs, do NOT leave exercise and nutrition out of your wellness equation. But, be advised that if they don't go to a gym now, they will not go if you give them a gym membership. However, if you place the exercise program in front of them, 45% - 75% of them will attend right out of the gate.

You do not need a fitness facility. You simply need a conference room or empty office and a Personal Fitness Trainer certified in training groups and special populations. Your on-site fitness programs must be directed by a Trainer who can work with multiple fitness levels simultaneously and write programming to progress everyone at their own pace.

Employees will work out on their lunch break or before or after work because it's convenient, there is peer support and encouragement, and there is a schedule and a plan that has considered their individual goals. The human body begins feeling and seeing the benefits of exercise immediately.

The Personal Fitness Trainer becomes as important to your business as your financial, legal, marketing, sales, production, and maintenance experts are. They help move your wellness program in the direction of prevention and healing and increase employee participation.

CEOs know that action is what turns the profit, fuels the growth, feeds the vision, and secures a healthier future. Is your company CEO in action with a mind for wellness?

So What's the Bottom Line?

Here are the cold, hard statistics for your unwell workforce:

- Presenteeism accounts for 61% of an employee's total lost productivity and medical costs.

- Employees working at diminished capacity cost employers over $250 billion a year. They cost you $2,000 to $2,800 per employee per year.

- Absenteeism costs an average of $789 per employee per year (as of 2002).

- Average cost of health insurance premium is $8,000 for employee-only, and $12,500 for employee with dependents. Wellness programs can net a 10% to 20% discount in these costs from the healthcare insurer.

- Average cost of absenteeism and presenteeism in a workforce is 10% of the compensation.

- Average cost of direct medical expenses is 7% of the compensation.

For assistance in calculating your own costs, you may find the Blueprint for Health helpful. It is free and available online. It is a service of the Health as Human Capital Foundation. Visit www.hhcfoundation.org/hhcf to register.

Implementing an effective wellness program can reduce these costs tremendously, including a 10% to 20% savings in health insurance premiums. Workers' Compensation premiums can be reduced. Direct medical costs, if you have a self-insured plan, will plummet. Absenteeism and presenteeism will be reduced dramatically.

Successful implementers of wellness programs indicate a return on investment ranging from $3 for every dollar spent to well over $5.

4

HOW DO CORPORATE WELLNESS PROGRAMS WORK?

Wellness programs run the gamut...as do success rates.

The most casual and inexpensive may include only online information and the occasional newsletter.

More common programs include HRAs (health risk assessments), some recommendations, and newsletters. They may also offer online support for diet management, or motivational tips for fitness.

The most robust and successful combine all of these elements and add, among other things, employee assistance programs, nutritional counseling, one-on-one coaching, on-site exercise programs, online support for exercising and nutrition, preventive care incentives, and incentives for desired behaviors. The possibilities are endless.

The main elements in any good wellness program include:

Management commitment. All successful wellness programs include involvement and commitment by management, from the top down.

Identification of risk factors. This identification can be achieved through HRAs, physicals, surveys, or any number of methodologies. The identification will generally stay private between the employee and whoever or whatever gathers the data. The employer is not privy to this information.

Recommendations to reduce risk factors. These recommendations may be generalized, or they may be customized to the employee, if they are arrived at through online systems or consultation with a healthcare provider.

Biological statistics. Some programs augment a health risk assessment with a basic health profile including body mass index, blood pressure, cholesterol levels, glucose levels, etc.

Goals and Incentives. To ensure achieving some kind of successful change in behaviors and the resultant health-related statistics, employees should be given, or should establish for themselves, some sort of goal. The goal can be to lose a certain number of pounds, to reduce cholesterol, to reduce blood pressure, etc. Incentives can be offered either for reaching the goal, or if the goal is not shared with the employer for privacy reasons, the incentive can be given for the employee taking the actions that would generally lead to the reaching of the goal. Conveniently, many goals can be reached by the simple tasks of stopping smoking, eating healthier, exercising more, and taking steps to manage stress. So there can be some generic activity goals that will qualify employees to receive incentives without the employer knowing too much detail about what their goals are.

Active Participation. The program will be only as effective as the employees allow it to be. As mentioned earlier, support from management (from the owner down) will go a long way to promoting employee participation. The adoption of a wellness culture where it becomes clear that a healthy, active, vital and vibrant workforce is a priority will also encourage participation. Any number of incentives for participation may be utilized as well. Contests, challenges, and active marketing of the program to the employees will also increase participation.

Multiple Touch-points. It's important that information, services and support for the program be made available to employees at times and in ways that are convenient for them. If you have an employee who would like to seek nutritional assistance at 9 p.m. online, it's helpful to have a program that has an interactive nutritional guide available on the website. If you have employees who prefer to read hard copy, printed materials should be available. Hotlines for consultation with a healthcare provider for those who like to speak with someone are also available. Online videos for education or exercise can be helpful to employees who are on the road or do most of their participation at home during off hours. Face-to-face support for nutritional counseling or exercise/fitness coaching can be invaluable in keeping employees engaged, educated and accountable.

Some of the less common variables that can be added include:

• Establishment of a wellness committee or leader

- Lunch and Learn programs

- Wellness information library

- Supporting community health effort

What's the relationship between wellness programs and your health insurance company?

Some programs are offered by health insurance companies. Others are provided by unrelated vendors. Sometimes health insurance companies work with outside vendors to deliver certain services.

If your health insurance company doesn't provide a wellness program of any kind, you will want to discuss potential future reductions in premiums with your agent. An insurance company that does not support wellness programs may not be willing to provide a discount. If that's the case, you may want to consider moving carriers to one that is more in line with your priorities.

If you have a self-insured health plan, your third party administrator (TPA) may provide services, or may be able to refer you to qualified vendors. Or, you may want to shop around for a vendor that's suitable, and then connect them with your TPA for administration.

Some workers compensation companies also offer loss prevention consulting and activities. Injury prevention activities can include such things as stretching at the desk to prevent carpal tunnel or back problems. Training on proper lifting, stress management, ergonomic workstations, proper posture, etc. can all minimize repetitive stress injuries and musculoskeletal injuries.

5

TRYING VERSUS DOING

Have you tried implementing a wellness program in the past and seen few, if any, positive results?

Don't let this stop you!

Because of the wide variety of new programs, the latest medical advances, and the prevalence of the internet in people's lives, there are many more choices for wellness programs.

In the past, many so-called wellness programs consisted merely of a health screening and monthly newsletters that employees wouldn't even bother to read. Programs today are much more sophisticated, but most importantly, they can be customized to your employees' needs and preferences.

If you do the groundwork up front to survey your employees, understand their concerns, their preferences for information delivery, and the level of participation they're willing to undertake, you can pick and choose the services needed, and the modes of communication.

What are the hallmarks of an ineffective program? Two common symptoms are lack of participation by employees, and lack of return on investment.

The most common reasons wellness programs fail to

achieve their desired goals are:

- Lack of employee interest

- Insufficient staff resources committed

- Insufficient funding committed

- Failure to engage high-risk employees

- Insufficient management commitment

These failure precursors are not listed in order of importance, and they frequently occur in combinations. Being aware of these obstacles can help you implement a successful program.

There are ways to neutralize each of these obstacles. Most of them can be avoided completely by thorough research of options, and by surveying employees to determine their needs and preferences prior to making your decisions about what and how to implement.

Lack of communication is one of the main reasons for employees not being interested in participating in a wellness program. Sometimes there are logistical issues, such as child care or transportation needs if the employee is to engage in a fitness activity before or after work. Other times the employee mistakenly believes an activity will cost money when it is included within the program. Or employees do not understand how the program will benefit them.

If lower level managers are in charge of disseminating information about the program to their staff, correct communication of the benefits of the program may be lacking.

Surveying employees prior to implementing a plan will allow you to identify those employees who are predisposed to participating in the plan. They can then be enlisted to help others understand the program and become motivated about participating. Some of these employees may also serve on a wellness program committee.

Unfortunately, some employees will be resistant to a program simply because they are upset with management or their supervisor, or because they believe the employer having an interest in their health is an invasion of their privacy. Only time and a track record of successful, healthy employees will have an influence on these people. In the interim, you will want to keep the positive communication high so their negative attitude does not impact the other motivated employees.

Dedicating staff resources to promoting and managing the wellness program is critical to the program's success. These staff resources should be personnel with experience in behavioral management, wellness and program design. The better versed they are in all aspects of wellness programs, the more successful they will be in communicating needed information, managing the program and evaluating its success. After the launch period, this work would not be a full-time job in most organizations.

Common Objections To Implementing Wellness Programs

By now, I hope you've come to see the need for a wellness program and how it could save you money in the long run, but you're still unsure whether you want to move forward. You're not alone. There are some common objections to implementing a wellness program, so lets review and overcome them.

1. "It's too expensive."

Programs can cost as little as $5 per employee. This type of program will consist largely of newsletter type informational support. No high-tech interactive programs, no screenings, no one-on-one coaching. Will this type of program do any good? Maybe. If your employees take the time to read the periodical information, they can benefit from various helpful tips to improve their health.

A mid-range program will cost perhaps $35 per employee per year. Keeping in mind again the $2,000 - $2,800 you lose for each employee operating at reduced productivity, an investment of $35 per employee doesn't seem like much, does it? If you can get just one or two employees on track with a mid-range program that offers information, several activities, and some interactive support, you will be well ahead of the game.

A top-drawer program might cost over $100 per employee per year. These programs may include screenings, personal coaching, nutritional advice, as well as interactive programs, wellness libraries, and periodical information.

2. "It takes too much time."

Not counting the time you expect your employees (and yourself) to invest in wellness activities, much of the time spent running a program happens during its initial establishment. Many wellness providers can handle a lot of the heavy lifting for you. They can survey employees, summarize and interpret results, recommend program structures, design communications, handle scheduling and sign-ups, create individualized programs and options, etc.

Although there is a lot of planning to be done, you do not have to do it all yourself.

Additionally, you will need to determine what constitutes an adequate return on investment for your program, and what metrics you will use to measure them. Once you have identified those two critical items, you will need to spend some time in the future evaluating your program. Again, your wellness program provider could provide services that will relieve you of the obligation to determine whether goals are being met. Only you, however, are suited to review results and determine if they are meeting the return on investment you have targeted.

How much time does this take? That depends on how much support you get from your provider, how many employees you have, and what kind and number of metrics you are measuring. It could take as little as an hour of review with your provider annually. Or it could be something you want your human resources manager to look at and report on monthly or quarterly, if you want to keep closer tabs on progress and participation.

To keep this time obligation in perspective, think about the amount of time you currently spend dealing with absenteeism, turnover and disciplinary issues in your company, and how much less time you will be spending once your wellness program takes hold. An investment of a few hours a year or quarter in maintaining a well-planned program will net significant returns.

3. "How do I know it will work?"

In the end, you cannot be absolutely certain that the wellness program will work until you implement it and look back a year or two down the road and see how much better your staff is performing and feeling. However, evidence abounds that a well-planned program is extraordinarily effective.

If you have the bad luck of having a few chronically ill people in your company who refuse to lift a finger to help themselves become healthier, no amount of wellness programs in the world will help you. However, most employers have a combination of people who are healthy, those who are middle-of-the-road but motivated to improve, those who are less healthy and will consider taking baby steps to improve, and those who are hard-core resistant to doing anything more at work than they absolutely must to collect a pay check.

A range of behavioral methods may be applied to get the

last group to participate in anything remotely related to a company benefit, especially one that requires their active engagement. Many will work. However, if this last group comprises only 10% of your workforce, you have a good probability of getting some participation out of the remaining 90%. If you do, you will see phenomenal results. Remember that on an average, less than 25% of the employee workforce participates once a week or more in a wellness program. Yet, the employers who have that level of participation say they get back between $3 and $5 for every dollar they invested in the program.

4. "It'll take too much effort to get a program up and running."

Again, here's where choosing the correct vendor is critical. If you don't have the staff resources or energy to put into establishing a new program, interview only those wellness experts who will do the "leg work" for you. You'll find that if you go online and search for "wellness programs" you'll have a good list of potential providers to interview very quickly.

Interviewing a few vendors is a good idea, but if you find that you don't have the tolerance for that process, speak to your business contacts. They may be able to provide a solid recommendation. Or, simply choose a company that offers programs customizable to the size of your organization, and then let them do the work of figuring out how to proceed.

The provider can then take over any complex and time-consuming tasks related to surveying employees, establishing baselines, coordinating with your healthcare insurance company, and so on.

Now that you know the reasons you need to consider implementing a wellness program, and you're familiar with all the things that don't work, let's talk about how you can make a positive, meaningful change in your workplace, and your employees' health and productivity.

PART TWO

THE SOLUTION

Management Commitment

If your workforce perceives a wellness program as a "do as I say, not as I do" offering from management, they won't be inclined to take advantage of it. If the inhabitants of the executive suite are fat, red-faced, and breathless after a short walk and do nothing to change that, the program, and the employer's commitment to it will be viewed as an exercise in hypocrisy.

Management must not only commit to the importance of the wellness program, a good proportion of executives, managers and supervisors must participate in the program to lead by example.

Solid Research and Planning

You must understand your employee population, their needs and propensities in order to choose a program that offers appropriate services and solutions for them. You must also research available programs to ensure you are selecting one that provides the flexibility, cost-effectiveness, and resources you and your employees need.

Employee Buy-in and Participation

Employees must understand the program, why it is necessary, how it will benefit them, and how to use it. You must find ways to motivate them to use the program and reward them for reaching certain goals.

Do not neglect yourself or other executives or management when thinking about motivation, rewards and incentives. Executives and management may be senior to the remainder of the staff in terms of corporate hierarchy, but may well be junior in terms of health, fitness, and wellness.

You may consider such incentive options as contests, a special parking space for the winner, a half-day off, "fitness bucks," recognition, massage gift certificates, etc. Use your creativity, and get feedback from the employees as to what will motivate them.

What Will Make Your Program Stellar?

To really kick your program up to the level where it will bring as many employees as possible under its spell and help them improve their health, vigor and productivity, there are a few more program characteristics that are essential.

Collaborative Team Support

People generally accept change better if they feel they've contributed to the decision-making that drives it. Your program will enjoy a more effective launch and more acceptance up front if trusted employee leaders (these are not always managers or supervisors but frequently line employees to whom others naturally look up) participate in the research, planning and development phases of the wellness program. This is much more effective than presenting staff with a finished product that they never saw coming. They will feel more connected to the process, and the program will have built-in advocates sprinkled throughout the company in strategic areas.

Another benefit of the collaborative approach is that the work required to launch and monitor the program will be shared among several people, rather than burdening one. The ability to obtain various perspectives is also valuable.

Expert Vendor Support

Some health insurance companies offer wellness programs (generally of a very limited variety). If you're going to take the next step and go beyond the minimal program your health insurance company may offer, then you will want a vendor with expertise and good support systems that dovetail with your main objectives.

A vendor with a human resources background and no fitness expertise, for example, will provide you with a different product than a vendor with healthcare and fitness professionals on staff. The optimal vendor needs to understand change implementation, corporate behavioral management, fitness, sports psychology, motivation, nutrition, health assessment protocols, confidentiality regulations, and a host of other disciplines.

Very few vendors have such broad expertise in-house, so it is quite common and appropriate for some services to be outsourced to other suppliers. Your vendor may continue to act as the point person and coordinator for the structuring of the program and the implementation of those portions in which they have expertise.

Measurable Goals

As with any corporate objective, you must establish your current benchmarks, identify the desired goals, and have a way to measure your progress.

If your short-term goal is to get your healthcare insurance costs down, you will want to find out what behaviors or activities can earn you premium credits with your company. If they don't offer any wellness program discounts, you might want to shop for another insurance company. In this case, the insurance company will dictate your goals.

If your goal is to get your direct healthcare costs down, or to minimize your on-the-job injuries, you will have somewhat different milestones and benchmarks.

If your goal is to maximize employee productivity and minimize absenteeism, again, your metrics will vary.

Your vendor will be able to assist you in determining what your true goals are, and in defining benchmarks, metrics and milestones so that you can track your progress.

On-Going Evaluations

You will need to establish a schedule upon which you will evaluate your progress to see if the program is having the desired results. If participation is low, you will address the motivation/reward/incentive model, or communication regarding the program and its benefits, or survey your staff to see what their issues with the program are.

If participation is good, you will want to determine if you're making progress on your goals pertaining to absenteeism, productivity, injuries, etc. Surveys, performance metrics, insurance company loss data, direct healthcare loss data (not individually identifiable, of course), all can provide such needed information.

Updates & Modifications

In addition to program changes needed to improve utilization or outcomes, there will often be new modalities, services or activities available which you will want to consider. If a program is getting stale, and participation is backsliding, you would want to offer new activities and/or services. You will want to do periodic surveys of participants and nonparticipants alike to see what their experience of the program is, or what their point of resistance is. As you adjust the program offerings to address these issues to the extent you can, you will see increased utilization and benefits.

7

HOW DO YOU FIND THE RIGHT PROGRAM?

There is a plethora of wellness programs available to you today. You can find them online, referenced in newsletters from your healthcare insurer, advertising in the newspapers, exhibiting at fitness fairs and wellness expos, and advertising at gyms. The choices can be overwhelming.

To guide you in determining what kind of vendor or program will work for you, ask yourself the following questions:

1. What are my main goals in pursuing a wellness program?

2. What kind of time and money am I willing to invest in developing and managing this program?

3. If my employees participate to the fullest, what kind of time will that take out of their days? What concessions am I willing to make, if any, during the work day for them to participate in wellness activities? This could include flexible lunch hours, flexible start or stop times to the work day, offering child care or commute assistance to expand the window during which an employee can engage in activities, and so on.

4. How much on-site, online, or phone support do I need to manage this program?

5. How much on-site, online, or phone support will my employees need to utilize the program?

6. Do I have staff on-hand who are familiar with wellness and motivated to lead the other employees in awareness and participation in the program?

7. Do I have facilities on-site that allow employees to engage in fitness activities without leaving the office? If not, do I need them, or is there an alternative?

8. Will my employees know a good thing when they see it and take advantage of this program? Or, will they need repeated motivation, solicitation, and perhaps even some hand-holding to participate regularly?

9. Will I need my vendor to provide face-to-face support and encouragement for me and my wellness team? To the employees?

Once you have answers to the above questions firmly in your mind, you will have an idea of the kind of support you need from a vendor, and this will help you choose the right one. From there, the vendor and you will determine the correct type of program for your company, including what services or activities will be offered, the frequency of those services or activities, and even what rewards or incentives might best be utilized.

How to Determine Your Program is Working

Only you will know what your goals are, but we know what

some common ones are, so let's review how you can determine the effectiveness of your program using some typical metrics.

Metabolic Syndrome Indicators

Whether you have a self-insured healthcare program or purchase commercial healthcare insurance, you will want to be aware of Metabolic Syndrome, and its risk factor indicators. This phrase is a recently coined buzzword that basically means the subject person suffers from a combination of enough particular risk factors that he is considered to be teetering on the edge of ill health.

The risk factors include:

- Elevated waist circumference
- Elevated triglycerides
- Reduced HDL ("good") cholesterol
- Elevated blood pressure
- Elevated fasting glucose

If a person has three of these five factors, he or she is considered to be at elevated risk for cardiovascular disease (heart attack, stroke, etc.) and/or Type 2 diabetes.

Since being overweight is commonly associated with high blood pressure and high cholesterol, you can imagine that it isn't much of a stretch to figure out there is a high percentage of overweight people who will have metabolic syndrome.

In addition to smoking cessation, the American Heart Association recommends the following steps to manage the risks associated with Metabolic Syndrome:

Weight loss, increased physical activity, and healthy eating habits.

Conveniently, a workplace wellness program can assist employees in doing each and every one of those things.

Your employees can be encouraged to have a health screening to determine their Metabolic Syndrome risk factors. The results of this screening will be completely confidential, but you, as the employer, can be advised what percentage of your staff is at risk.

After implementation of a wellness program, these screenings can be repeated periodically, and you can enjoy seeing the percentage of at-risk staff reduced over time. The reduction of the risk factors will mean less likelihood of incidents of ill health, absenteeism and medical costs for your staff and your company.

Injury Statistics

If you have a workforce that's large enough to negate the impact of "bad luck" on the data, you can get strong evidence of the success of a wellness program in terms of job-site injuries.

For example, if you have a large workforce, especially if the workforce is in an industry prone to injury, such as construction trades, you will have extensive injury data from your workers' compensation carrier (or your third party administrator if you're self-insured, where that is an option). After implementation of a wellness program, and controlling for other safety measures or training that may have been implemented in the same time period, you will be able to see that your workers with stronger, healthier, more alert and focused bodies and minds are not getting injured on the job as often as they used to be.

Healthcare Cost Statistics

You will never know exactly who has what ailment or whether they are recovering, unless that employee chooses to share the information with you.

What you can know is what your overall staff looks like in terms of risk factors, if your employees participate in screening, and utilization of services – both preventative and allopathic.

If you purchase commercial insurance, check with your healthcare insurance company and find out what steps you can take and what programs you can implement that will gain you an immediate discount in your premium. If your agent or carrier has an answer to that inquiry, you can bet your bottom dollar that they have found those steps and programs to be very beneficial to them in reducing utilization. What is beneficial for them will be beneficial to you.

After you have implemented your program, you can review utilization over various time periods, and health screening data (again, this data will be aggregated and not individually identifiable, but still helpful), and determine whether your program is succeeding in achieving your objectives. Your health insurance carrier may only discount your premium for certain activities or metrics, but you will gain continued and additional benefits due to reduced absenteeism, presenteeism, and increased focus and vitality or your workers.

If you have a self-insured program, you can work with your Third Party Administrator (TPA) to determine the same information, and more importantly, once you have chosen a wellness program vendor, they can work with your TPA to coordinate results and program revisions. For every single dollar not needed for healthcare, you will enjoy a direct return on your investment. You may find that the preventative care expenditures increase a bit as your employees become more interested in their health and wellness. But as we all know, most serious illnesses are significantly less expensive to treat when they are caught early, versus when they have ravaged the body and caused catastrophic disruption in the employee's life.

Improved Productivity and Attendance

Absenteeism, sick days, time off for doctor's appointments, late arrivals, and other indicators of ill health, presenteeism and a distracted workforce will be greatly reduced after the implementation of an effective program.

These metrics are easy enough to measure if you have been tracking them prior to implementation of your wellness program. If you did not previously monitor these statistics, you might find it helpful to start tracking them at the beginning of the program, then check them quarterly. Your first quarter will be somewhat improved from statistics prior to implementation, but the benefits will not yet have matured, so you will see continued improvement for several months, if not years.

Increased Camaraderie and Employee Morale

One of the "soft" benefits of a successful wellness program is increased esprit de corps and loyalty in the employee ranks. As staff participates in wellness activities together and begin to see benefits, supporting each other in their successes, and assisting each other with challenges, they create a common ground that otherwise would not exist. Employees who hardly speak to each other during the work day due to divergent responsibilities can develop strong bonds through shared wellness activities.

Increased morale is a more difficult outcome to measure than the "hard" benefits mentioned above. One of the best ways to gauge it is to have the wellness team members informally survey employs on a periodic basis. Honest communication regarding loyalty and morale is notoriously challenging when employers ask their employees direct questions pertaining to such matters. However, if trusted colleagues ask less direct questions and pay careful attention to the grapevine and people's behavior and interactions, they can provide valuable information.

Benefits of increased morale and loyalty include less turnover and higher productivity, so although they are difficult to measure, they are desirable goals.

Increased Employee Perception Of Employer Engagement

Employees of organizations providing wellness programs routinely cite the program as evidence that the employer cares about their well-being. Loyalty being a two-way street, a program is a very effective way to show your employees that they are important to you, and they tend to return the sentiment. Employers reap tremendous economic benefits from implementing an effective wellness program, and the prospect of obtaining those benefits is usually the initial motivating factor in pursuing a program. However, employers generally also take into consideration the humanitarian motivation of wanting to do something to improve the lives of your employees.

To the extent you are implementing the program because your employees will benefit from it, your employees will tend to recognize that level of caring and will reciprocate.

This again is a "soft" benefit and not easily quantified. However, it can be gauged by use of anecdotal evidence and information gathering.

8

WHAT DOES YOUR PERFECT PROGRAM LOOK LIKE?

Is there one perfect wellness program that works for every company, every time? No, there is not. However, you can create a wellness program that is perfect for your company and your employees.

Many corporate wellness programs have fallen short of this perfect wellness program scenario. The good news is that they don't have to stay stuck where they are and they don't have to throw in the towel. Chances are that program was a mixture of insurance and employee benefit provider options with a few other components added in for good measure in the premise that something will work.

Many of those companies whose wellness programs have fallen short of their perfect ideal understand the value of taking time to investigate what their customers want and need and trying to out-market their competition to boost their profits. When a company applies a similar process to their employee wants and needs for wellness and understands the competition for wellness, they can create an effective foundation on which to build their perfect wellness program.

With numerous vendors at your fingertips who can provide a large variety of expertise, services, resources, and activities for any and every aspect of your wellness program, how do you know which one or combination is perfect for you?

If you have a program in place that is not working for you, simply step back for a moment to consider a "do over."

Let's take a brief look at something here. You create awareness among your employees of company policies, give them clear job descriptions, and explain their role in their position, their department, and the company as a whole. Then you educate them by telling and showing them their job and all the elements and activities they will be doing on a daily, weekly, and monthly basis.

Does it stop there? No. The employee now has to DO their job. All of the awareness and education about their job you provide will be of no use to you or them if they do not DO their job.

How do you facilitate that action? You provide the tools, the location, and the guidance that is required for them to DO their job. Plus, you pay them for it.

Once your employees become aware of their health status and are educated as to what they must be doing to change their health status for the better, only a handful of those employees will have enough initiative to follow through and take action by themselves.

When you provide the tools, location, and the guidance that is required for them to DO wellness, they will DO wellness.

When they don't have to find their own way and traverse the myriad of obstacles and barriers that come at them each day, when the path is paved and the way is clear, the employees who gave input and feel listened to, will participate, and will get well.

The human body and the human mind, though very complex, are also very predictable. Working with it you can achieve success. Working against it, any success is very short-lived and minimal.

Twenty different companies can use this same identical process and wind up with very similar, yet very different perfect wellness programs. The beauty of this plan is that it works for every business and every company that implements it.

Disease management with medications cannot give you the same results. With much research now showing prescription drugs as the fourth leading cause of death in America, can your business afford not to address the lifestyle causes of chronic illness? Can your business afford to simply hand off gym memberships to employees and tell them "Go to it!" when 70% - 80% of them won't go anyway? Can your business afford to feed the poor nutrition habits of fast food lunches and vending machine fats and calories?

When you create an environment that sustains your well-thought-out wellness program foundation and framework, you will see a natural gravitation toward wellness that becomes infectious throughout your company, increasing your productivity and profits. And that, after all, is the heart of your perfect wellness program.

Because there is such variety in vendors and the expertise, services, resources and activities they offer, there's no telling exactly what your program will look like. However, there are certain attributes it is likely to have, and there is a very broad menu of services and activities from which you are likely to choose.

Here are the attributes your successful program will have:

Efficiency

Your program will be efficient. You will see results with an appropriate amount of effort. This pertains to your corporate effort and results, as well as the individual participant's effort and results. The program will be designed to meet your needs so that you're not spending money on things you don't utilize or value. Some programs will provide results within 12 weeks so you can quickly evaluate them.

Expertise

Your program will be developed by qualified persons. Those providers will exercise ongoing oversight to ensure that you are offered the latest technology and science.

Timing

Your program will provide for information and resources to

be accessed at times that are convenient for you and your employees. There will also be sufficient time blocked out during, before or after the work day for people who want to participate to do so.

Flexibility

Your program will allow for services to be utilized and activities to be undertaken at times and places that are convenient for you and your employees. This may mean group exercise classes on-site or in a nearby facility or park, and those classes may be before, after or during work, depending on your facilities.

Online training videos, online or face-to-face nutritional counseling or exercise programming can be used any time of the night or day. Audio training, iPod downloads, and other current technology delivery systems will ensure the highest level of flexibility.

Effective and Cost-effective

Your program will be effective. You will see measurable results. It will also be cost-effective. Cost will be variable based on the services you utilize. Some activities or services may be paid for in part by the employees.

Your provider is so committed to the success of your program that they will create or contribute to financial incentives such as charging you only for those employees who participate or providing bonus money to the employee who wins a performance or weight loss contest.

Informative

Your program will include necessary and helpful information. This includes education of the management team, including all executives from the top down. Employee education as to the importance of wellness and the features, services, resources and activities of the program will also be provided. There will be a library of resource materials, available on-site, or online. On-site Lunch 'n' Learns will be offered on a periodic basis, quarterly (or more frequent) newsletters will be provided, and periodic emails directly to employees will disseminate helpful tips regarding fitness and nutrition.

There will be a feedback loop so the wellness team can monitor progress and participation and recommend adjustments or additions to the program.

9

A CASE STUDY

The following is an overview of the delivery systems, protocols and successes of the AYC Corporate Wellness System.

AYC's Corporate Wellness System is an outgrowth of AYC Health & Fitness, a Kansas City-based fitness organization dedicated to fitness and health for over 30 years.

AYC's clients range from small organizations, to large, publicly-traded companies. Costs per employee vary, depending on class size and number of programs AYC delivers.

A key component to AYC's success, and the success of each client, is that AYC brings the wellness program to the client. We don't sell the program and remain passively on the sidelines while the client does or does not implement the program successfully.

After assessing the needs of each company through management and employee interviews and surveys, we create a personalized program. AYC provides each company with all the tools needed to implement the program, and we provide on-site exercise sessions and consultations with individuals regarding optimal exercise programs. Nutritional counseling is referred to registered dietitians. Health screenings are also made available through outside resources.

AYC handles most administrative paperwork for the employer, as well as assisting the HR department in handling the promotion of the program to the employees.

A program is initially instituted for a test period of three months. Baseline measurements and statistics are recorded for all participating employees at the beginning of that time, and results are recorded after the 12-week period has concluded. AYC has been successful in persuading participants to "put their money where their mouth is," and if a participating employee sees no benefit at the end of the 12-week period, he must reimburse the employer for part of his or her program costs - which very rarely happens. Dedication by the employees to achieving results has skyrocketed due to a shared commitment by the company and AYC.

Busy executives or other staff members who travel frequently need not feel left out. Unique online exercise programs keep traveling employees on track and in training even while on the road. Exercises may be accessed via the internet, or downloaded onto an iPod. Many exercise programs are devised for body-weight resistance, and do not need weights or gym equipment to be effective.

Online resources also include exercise-tracking logs, meal planners for weight loss, muscle building, performance improvement, or just about any other goal the employee might have. There is also a meal diary application to allow each participant to track calories consumed and a grocery list for suggested meal plans.

Due to time constraints shared by many companies, AYC has developed high-intensity 30 minute workouts that may be conducted before work or during lunch, if the employer has showering facilities, or after work without undue disruption to the employees' commutes. These workouts are commonly held in small groups from 10 to 15 employees, and can be performed in a small area such as a conference room, or a larger facility such as an on-site gym or a cafeteria. This flexibility is one of the keys to the program's success.

The personal interaction and attention from the AYC team is also a major factor that ensures the individual employee's (and employer's) success with the program. AYC remains actively involved in the administration and implementation of every aspect. They assist in conducting the pre-program surveys of employees and help the employer determine the likelihood of participation by their employees, and the correct types of services and activities to offer.

The AYC team is in contact with the employer throughout the entire 12-week introductory period, consults with employees as needed, and communicates with all enrollees via email with health and nutritional tips.

After the initial 12-week period, AYC evaluates the program's success to date, and makes any needed adjustments. Employees evaluate their improvements and set new goals. Subsequent cycles are run in eight-week intervals, and the program is re-evaluated and adjusted as needed at the end of each cycle. The program is promoted to engage additional enrollees, and they are incorporated into the system as quickly and seamlessly as possible.

AYC clients have enjoyed an average weight loss of nine pounds during the initial 12-week period, and an increase in aerobic fitness of over 15%. Employers have noted that absenteeism has dropped and energy levels have increased. Employees are happier and more productive. The program has also become a selling point for new hires.

AYC's Critical Success Components:

- Capturing CEO support

- Designating a company wellness leader or team

- Conducting an employee health interest survey

- Providing an opportunity for health screening

- Administering an annual physical activity campaign

- Holding a nutrition Lunch and Learn sessions

- Establishing an in-house wellness library

- Creating email newsletters

- Implementing health policies and procedures

- Supporting community health efforts

- Active engagement of the provider with the employees

AYC is a full-service provider that creates and implements a customized program and provides the employer with every possible chance at succeeding in attaining their program goals.

10

NINE TRUTHS ABOUT WELLNESS PROGRAMS

I hope by this point you've come to realize that most of the hype and complicated information you've seen about wellness programs is nothing but lies and myths.

The truth is that implementing an effective and successful program boils down to two main elements: Committing to the goal, and picking an appropriate partner. (This holds true in business, sports, and marriage too!)

So, let's take another look at the lies and myths, only this time in mirror image, now that you have the truth to rely upon:

1. Healthcare costs are going up, and you can do a lot to control your employees' need for medical attention.

2. Your employees' health is very much your business, as it impacts their productivity, their performance, and their co-workers.

3. People get sick, and a great deal of that sickness is preventable and due to lifestyle choices.

4. The right wellness program is not only affordable, it's cost-effective and provides up to 10 times the return on investment.

5. The administration of a wellness program can be

delegated to the right provider.

6. Solid benefits for wellness programs have been researched for over 20 years, and they have been proven time and again.

7. You don't need extensive facilities for your employees to gain the benefits of exercise.

8. Many of your employees will want to participate, and there are many ways to motivate those who are on the fence.

9. It's easy to establish and measure goals and results from the program.

Now that you know the TRUTH about wellness programs, what are you waiting for?

Start your search for a provider TODAY! Get the ball rolling and survey your employees. Do not waste another day waiting for your employees (and yourself) to be drowned in the tidal wave of ill health that is washing over our population, and could eventually kill your business.

PART THREE

RESOURCES

AVERAGE WELLNESS TO REVOLUTIONARY WELLNESS IN ONLY THREE MONTHS...

Your Step-By-Step Guide To A Successful Corporate Wellness Program

The Old Wellness Program Model

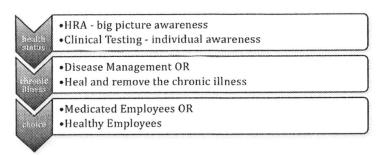

- **health status**
  - HRA - big picture awareness
  - Clinical Testing - individual awareness
- **chronic illness**
  - Disease Management OR
  - Heal and remove the chronic illness
- **choice**
  - Medicated Employees OR
  - Healthy Employees

The Big Question...Are they getting well?

Problem #1

CEO has not supported, endorsed, or participated in creating a sustainable wellness culture.

Without this support, there will be few followers of the wellness program and it will fall by the wayside. By introducing the wellness program as a ready-made "benefit" without employee input, the culture of the workplace leans toward compliance and feelings of intrusion. The natural tendency is not to embrace something that is forced on us, especially if it seems to apply to some and not all.

Without employee participation, health doesn't change and the program is deemed a failure.

Problem #2

Most businesses do not take advantage of all the benefits

they are paying for from their providers.

With little direction, communication, activities and events, momentum is lost. Insurance providers have a multitude of services and communication pieces in their arsenal, yet most won't volunteer them unless they are asked.

Problem #3

Most businesses do not know what it takes to get their employees healthy again.

Employees have human bodies and human bodies have specific requirements to regain and retain good health. Yes, chronic illness has everything to do with unhealthy lifestyle choices. Managing the chronic illness with medication does little to help activate healthy lifestyle changes or employee accountability.

Problem #4

Most businesses realize that regular exercise plays a role in achieving good health and leaves it up to the employee to make the time, and motivate themselves to get to a gym.

When an individual has never worked out or been inside a gym in their entire life, we are talking about a major lifestyle change. Giving them a discount at a local gym is tantamount to giving them a book written in Greek and asking them to give you a book report in three months. Will they be able to do it?

No.

Without regular exercise, the chronic illness does not improve. Reassessment measures show no improvement, and the program is called a failure.

Problem #5

Offering information and education only, with no challenge, incentive, or drive toward attainable healthy lifestyle choices.

Most people know when they are choosing something that is not good for them. Many people have a difficult time changing lifestyle behaviors because they are connected emotionally or mentally to previous rewards. If simple education and information was enough to facilitate a change to healthy choices, there would be no need for a wellness program.

A smoking cessation program that ends there without incorporating alternate healthy choices in the previous environment has limited success. Once again, the burden is unsupported lifestyle change completely on the shoulders of the employee.

AYC K.I.S.S. Model

Keep **I**ntegrating **S**imple **S**teps
in the Employee Wellness Environment

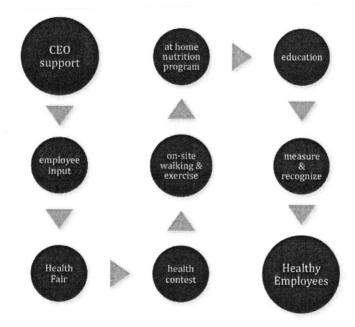

The **AYC K.I.S.S. Employee Wellness Environment** is supportive and systematic, with preparation and activation of healthy lifestyle choices that result in greater employee willingness and accountability for their own health.

K.I.S.S. your employees today using this wellness model and you will see startling and progressive healthy lifestyle changes in just three months.

Already have a lukewarm wellness program in place? AYC

can help you seamlessly integrate the **Smart K.I.S.S.** into your corporate culture

Smart K.I.S.S. #1

A letter of support from the CEO to each employee.

CEO support and participation is paramount to success. Introduce the concept and rationale behind the introduction of a wellness program and ask for employee input in developing the program.

Set the tone for your wellness program by openly and boldly providing an announcement and expression of support in the form of a personal letter to each employee from the CEO.

A letter that warmly embraces the employees, their contribution and value to the company, concern for their concerns, one that shares their hopes and dreams of quality life and a bright future…and asks for their input by means of a survey.

This preparation is paramount to helping employees take ownership of their wellness program and building desire and accountability for their own health.

When the CEO asks their opinions and thoughts and then acts on them by implementing some of those suggestions, the CEO establishes the credibility and supportive nature of the program.

When the CEO becomes noticeably healthier, supports and

recognizes the efforts of employees, they will follow and participate willingly, creating a culture of support, encouragement, and self-motivation among themselves.

Key point: If the CEO is obviously not making efforts to improve his or her own health, the letter will serve as a double standard to the employees. This negates the value of the letter, its message, and the wellness program. CEO support is the most critical element of all.

Smart K.I.S.S. #2
Designate a company wellness leader.

This may initially be the HR Director, or an enthusiastic employee who is willing to pick up the ball and run with it. We work with our clients (and their broker) to develop the timelines and programs that their employees want and need.

As your wellness program progresses and develops, team members and committees can be formed to distribute the responsibility and planning – no need to create a stressful situation of complete responsibility for any one individual.

Create the opportunity and the means for employees to participate in the planning and implementation of specific elements of your wellness program and you will see those employees mature in their self confidence and leadership ability.

Depending on the depth of the team leader responsibility, it may be worthwhile to build the time into that person's job description – again showing the high value the CEO places on the wellness program.

> ***With An Eye on the Big Picture*** *- Prior to or during these first two steps, the development of a Vision/Mission Statement (one or two sentences that declare your objectives for your company wellness program) and Goals/Objectives (written outline) will provide an excellent frame of reference and starting point.*

Smart K.I.S.S. #3
Conduct an employee health interest survey.

Before you introduce any elements of your wellness program, it will benefit you to conduct an employee health interest survey. All the basic elements you would introduce anyway will be included in the employee answers. Why not let all wellness activities and events be introduced after the employees are asked their opinions and needs by survey. Introducing any specific elements prior may be viewed with suspicion and inferred compliance.

We have attached our recommendations for survey questions along with standard questions that give the most input to developing a program that will be utilized and embraced by employees.

> **_With An Eye on the Big Picture_** - *After the Employee Health Interest Survey results are tabulated and the employee interests are obvious, it becomes imperative to generate roles and responsibilities for some of these projects. From the people who expressed desire for involvement, hold a meeting and fill the roles, define the responsibilities, and set timelines.*
>
> *The first order of business will be to establish baseline health measures with biometric screening and plan the elements of the health fair and introduction to the wellness program. You will want to get pricing for each element you wish to include and develop a budget to help with planning.*

Smart K.I.S.S. #4

Provide an opportunity for health screening.

A health fair is an ideal place to introduce the scope of your basic wellness program and offer employees a biometric screening. It would also give them the opportunity to participate in an health risk assessment if they desire. They could learn about resources that are available to them, such as intervention programs, lunch and learns, and educational seminars. In addition, you can provide specific information about key components of health and wellness, and have local experts talk about the prevention of common chronic illnesses.

An introduction to physical exercise and healthy nutrition

are key elements to keeping the body healthy. Be sure to include some type of physical activity for employees, and have nutritious food available for sampling.

A health fair can be perceived as a fairly safe place to explore wellness in the safety of the masses without calling much attention to one self. It can be a fun and interactive event that fuels enthusiasm.

__With An Eye on the Big Picture__ - Communicating your wellness program is an on-going process and ideally communication that takes many different forms will drive the message home more effectively. Newsletters, posters, emails, announcements, even newspaper recognition articles of special achievement, are all effective communication measures.

Smart K.I.S.S. #5
Administer an annual physical activity campaign.

Getting the employees involved in physical activity is imperative. Not all employees will join a regular exercise program at the start. By offering yearly physical activity campaigns, non-participating employees have a chance to take part and become engaged – and perhaps enjoy it enough to join a regular group activity.

Whether taking part in a community challenge, creating an internal department or sister company competition, or a special incentive challenge, something new should be offered once a year to pique interest of non-participants and give regular participants something more to strive for.

> *With An Eye on the Big Picture- Program evaluation and measurement are important. Decide what and how you will measure success. Use your goals and objectives to determine this. You could do evaluations after each major event such as a health fair or a yearly physical activity challenge, and for specific events every three to six months for regular exercisers. You can create separate time-tables for those with serious chronic illness, or anyone who prefers a 6-week reassessment.*

Smart K.I.S.S. #6
Hold Lunch-and-Learns.

Make a list of specific topics that were most requested on the employee survey. These will become some of your mainstay sessions that you will hold once a year, or bring back by popular demand.

Lunch and learn allows the opportunity for employees to experience healthy foods they may not be familiar with, and to listen to a topic of interest in a pleasant environment. The company also saves some time by holding these sessions over the lunch hour. Quarterly sessions are ideal.

Have the employees complete a survey after each lunch and learn to assess the value they placed on the topic, what they will do with the information they learned, the quality of the speaker, etc. We have attached a sample survey for this purpose.

Smart K.I.S.S. #7
Establish a company wellness library.

Educated and well-informed employees who have opportunity to participate in activities that generate health will want to know more. The more accurate health information they see and hear, the more likely they are to continue investigating and participating.

Your wellness library can contain information from reputable sources in the form of self-care books and health magazines, instructional DVDs, audio books, newsletters, pamphlets, and behavior change guides. With a few comfortable chairs nearby for easy reading and listening, and the ability to borrow material, more employees will utilize your wellness library.

Smart K.I.S.S. #8
Send out a quarterly health newsletter.

Health information distributed on a regular basis can create top of mind awareness. By offering a variety of topics, information will always be fresh and timely. Writing for a sixth grade level is a common practice for easy absorption and reading by all.

An article tied in with a quiz helps readers grasp more of the article, and completed quizzes may be used for a random drawing for special items – dinner for two at a healthy restaurant allows the winner to share their good fortune and the concept of health with someone close to them.

We have attached a list of thought starter topics that can be used in a health and wellness newsletter. We would be happy to submit a regular column. You may also wish to have a medical column with a guest physician each quarter, such as a chiropractor, women's health, men's health, internist, etc.

One column of the newsletter may also be devoted to the monthly calendar of national awareness (i.e.: February is National Heart Month), perhaps include a recipe (and employee comments about the previous recipe submitted). Success stories can be featured. Employees will begin seeing definite healthy changes in just a few short weeks.

Smart K.I.S.S. #9
Implement health promoting policies.

Policies and procedures that are written into a policy manual will become incorporated more easily in the workplace. Policies regarding health and safety that tie directly to state or federal laws and objectives of the company wellness program are appropriate for the policy manual.

Examples include the use of seat belts, safety and emergency procedures during a disaster, routine scheduling of first aid box inspection and refilling. Policies that tie directly to lifestyle choices might include a tobacco-free workplace and an alcohol/drug-free workplace.

Smart K.I.S.S. #10

Promote Community Health Efforts

Communities offer many health related events such as run/walk events, cycling events, health fairs and educational seminars that can be promoted and shared with your employees. From a business perspective, being active in the community and helping promote the community generates a feeling of goodwill toward the company. Your employees will benefit by being kept in the loop and encouraged to participate.

Many community events are covered in the media with film footage and photos. As your employees get coverage at these events, the excitement continues to build.

Sample Participant Survey (after Lunch-&-Learn)

Seven Keys to a Vibrant and Healthy Body

1. Was this Lunch-&-Learn a good experience for you? __Yes __No

2. What interested you the most?

_____

3. What changes do you plan on making in your life because of this experience?

_____

4. How often would you like to exercise?

___3 days per week. ___2 days per week. ___Not sure. ___None.

5. If you could participate in an exercise program at work, what time is best for you?

___ Before work. ___ Lunch time. ___ After work.

6. What other types of physical fitness activities interest you?

_____

7. What other topics are you interested in hearing about?

___ Walking ___ Bicycling ___Running ___Yoga ___Pilates

___ Strength & Toning ___ Cardio & Endurance

___ Flexibility / Range Of Motion / Stretching

___ How-to create lifestyle changes, one step at a time

___ Managing low back pain & stress reduction

___ Calories, nutrition & weight control

___Food labels - how to read / what to look for

___ Water / Sodas / Energy Drinks / Juices - What's healthy?

Other

_____

8. Did the speaker hold your interest, speak professionally, and know his/her material?

_____

9. Any changes you'd make to the presentation? Other topics not covered?

_____

Wellness Newsletters – Some Theme Ideas

Theme 1 - Perspectives
- Eating for nutrition, not to fill a rumbling stomach
- Exercising for health and mobility, not drudgery
- Mind/Body awareness, decisions and choices

Theme 2 - Exercise While You Wait
- Standing in the checkout line - stretch, twirl, move, etc.
- Sitting in the waiting room, or at your desk
- Fidget to burn calories -

Theme 3 - Buddy Body Moves
- Play with your kids, your spouse, your family and friends get out there and be active
- Walk or run with your dog
- Try a group bicycling ride

Theme 4 - Walk This Way
- Warm up before you walk
- Find ways to walk daily - park further away, etc.
- Stats on walking, 2,000 steps is a mile, 10,000 steps per day recommended

Theme 5 - Latest Startling Statistics
- From the news
- Prevention ideas
- Exercise and nutrition studies

Theme 6 - Exercise Tips
- Keep balance in your moves, work your bi's AND your tri's
- Supplement your workouts with other physical activities

Theme 7 - Personal Development
- Lifestyle choices
- Lead by example
- New body, new personality...better health, better outlook
- Creating healthy habits

Theme 8 - Little Things Matter
- Don't forget fingers, toes, wrists and ankles
- Do you really need that extra piece, that extra sitcom? Try something else instead.
- Goals

Theme 9 - Stretching
- Stretch only to the point of tension, not pain
- 2 second stretch prior to workout, longer stretch after body is warm

Theme 10 - Nutrition
- Use a nutrition system
- Eating clean
- Portion control

Theme 11 - Body Basics
- Stress reduction exercises and tips
- Low back pain relief
- The heart is a muscle too
- 3,500 calories = 1 lb. of fat, therefore 100 calories per day not burned...

Theme 12 - Preparation
- Shoes are made for walking...tips on proper footwear

- Buddy system for long distance training, hiking, etc.
- Know your exercising heart rate

Theme 13 - Personal Best
- Gaining health and losing weight and chronic illness, one step at a time
- Winners are those who....
- Motivational Quotes, applied to their corporate group
- Commendations, group totals for the quarter (get permission before featuring any individuals)

There are many more ideas not listed here. The possibilities are almost endless. More topics include: healthy recipes, holiday menus, vitamins and supplements, community health events calendar, health stats and warning signs of illness, and prevention of chronic illness. A newsletter is also an ideal place to post winners of challenges and event and program announcements.

How To Implement Effective Corporate Fitness Into Any Workplace

Times have changed yet the human body still has the same needs it had a thousand years ago.

The heart is still a muscle that needs regular exercise. The brain still needs an influx of fresh oxygen daily. The body still needs natural food for nourishments, and the bones, joints, and muscles still need regular exercise to stay healthy and well.

When the body does not receive the regular exercise and proper nutrition it needs, deterioration and chronic illness will thrive and can create disabilities, a drain on finances, time, energy, and dreams, as well as a premature death that was wholly preventable...with regular exercise and proper nutrition.

The simplest and most direct route to good health and wellness is the easiest and most rewarding to implement, from my experience. There are many, many reasons our country is experiencing a drastic decline in health and rapidly increasing costs associated with that declining health.

There is really only one reason that the simple and direct route is the road less traveled. That reason is lack of understanding. People, who survive a first heart attack and then are told by their doctor they MUST exercise regularly and start eating nutritious food or they will die, suddenly become alert with complete understanding. They can suddenly break down the barriers they felt they had and just as suddenly fit regular exercise and proper nutrition into their daily lives.

Let me show you how you, your employees, and your company don't have to get to the brink of death or financial drain before you take the action that reverses and prevents the majority of the reasons you are offering or considering a wellness program.

I invite you to explore the path that I have laid out before you in this report. Ask yourself the hard questions. Take another look at your employees and your corporate environment with fresh eyes.

This program, or one just like it, is totally doable for any company. Some companies may need modifications in scheduling, locations, or other factors, and all of that is workable. You can achieve healthy and productive employees who thrive on helping build a healthier and more profitable company when their bodies, minds, and spirits are fed and fueled as they were designed to be.

Let's take a look at the human body, which all of your employees have, without exception.

Survival of the Fittest

In the early days of human existence the average work day consisted of lifting and carrying heavy rocks, downed trees, and water, plowing and tilling the ground, and building fences and shelters. Travel was walking, running, or riding on an animal. The ground was uneven offering a multitude of physical obstacles to traverse, building strong bones and muscles, hearts and lungs.

The bottom line in the early days of human existence was if you don't work, you don't eat. You won't be sheltered, and you won't survive. Work was pushing, pulling, dragging, walking, running, lifting, and bending.

The human body is designed with joints and limbs to act as levers and they need maintenance the same as any machine with moving parts does. They also need regular use to avoid deterioration of their parts.

Health in the early days of mankind was at the whim of the seasonal food supply, which was harvested from the earth, natural and unadulterated. Early death was usually the cause of acute illness such as pneumonia or plague.

The natural cycles and rhythms of the human body were followed with sleep during darkened hours, rising with the sun, breathing fresh air, with increased oxygen uptake during working activities. All the ingredients of a well body were provided: fresh air, sunshine, stress reduction, regular exercise, proper nutrition, sleep, and water.

Mankind Redefines Survival of the Fittest (but the human body is still the same)

With the advent of the Industrial Age flowing into the Information Age, we have created a society where we sit passively at desks all day determined to prosper financially, quickly and with the least effort. Survival of the Fittest has been redefined as 'he who has the most toys wins'.

We no longer fight to survive the elements of nature and the needs of daily living. Our shelter and our food now come from others whom we simply exchange money with...the money we earn working for others, sitting at a desk or workstation all day

Our bodies are now challenged by a different set of physical activities. The strain of forward head and shoulders, weakened backs, stooping spinal columns, flabby leg muscles and too- tight hamstrings all contribute to defective postures, giving rise to aches, pains, stiffness, and compensation of limbs and joints that cause further deterioration and injury in the body too often at rest.

Who are the Fittest in Our Society?

The ones with the biggest house, the flashiest car, the most money? If you were to ask that question of a wealthy person, owner of the most riches in the world, who was flat on their back in the midst of pain and disability due to chronic illness, what do you suppose their answer would be?

While it is probably true that early man aspired to have more wealth, more land, more cows, the majority of them probably simply wanted to make a good life for their family in a way that reduced hardship. Perhaps it is the word "hardship" that we have redefined in our mind.

The "honest toil of working hands" has come to mean something so very different than early mankind could ever imagine. Fingers on a keyboard have replaced the process of putting your whole body weight behind the shovel and pushing then lifting the earth to move it, making way for a better future with more healthy crops.

Now we use our fingers and our brains – the new "brawn" of the 21st century. Fingers and brains can help our finances survive. They can help us in many ways, but they fall seriously short in the area of providing health and wellness to our bodies. The increased time spent sitting or using repetitive movements without balancing opposing structures creates a stress on our bodies as well as our minds. Increased stress, along with a sedentary lifestyle, begins a spiraling cycle in the downturn of health.

One of the most commonly asked questions I get is, "how can I receive the benefits of exercise without moving my body?" How can you earn interest on a savings account you never opened?

You can't.

Today it is commonly recognized that those who achieve good health, happiness, and productivity the most, are the ones who achieve physical fitness, mental fitness, and social fitness. Our society is so far removed from understanding how our bodies work and what its needs are. In addition, the word 'fitness' in our society has the basic perception of purpose to mean trim and sexy bodies.

Our fruitfulness and well-being are directly linked to the state of our health and while our bodies are very resilient and hardy, they have at the same time a delicate balance and require care. The world of business is about pursuing possibilities and growing great things. A healthy body feeds an active and productive mind capable of so much more than the weakened and hindered productivity level produced by acute or chronic illness and medicated minds and bodies.

The Human Body – The Bottom Line:

Your body has dynamic and powerful self-healing mechanisms that are fueled by vitamins, amino acids, and fatty acids.

That means that when you eat nutritious, natural food you give your body the tools it needs to repair and heal its self.

Systems that depend on this nutritious food for fuel include:

- Your brain chemistry
- Inflammation levels
- Digestion and elimination
- Blood cell quality
- Blood flow
- Concentration
- Sleep

Your bone and muscle system requires regular use, especially since your lymphatic flow completely depends on regular muscle contraction to function.

Your lymph system is part of your immune system, helping defend against disease and sickness.

Without regular exercise and proper nutrition, your body slowly breaks down into a state of disease.

Greg Justice, MA and Alicia Johnson, NMD have compiled this information to help you understand the importance of a lifestyle that includes regular exercise and proper nutrition.

The Foundation of Your Corporate Wellness Program

There are many reasons any given business will implement and offer a wellness program to their employees. Most of the rationale centers on saving time and money, and sometimes comes bundled with the leader's compassion of "it's the right thing to do."

When we look more closely at the "why" we can more effectively design for ROI impact in the "do."

Did your company leadership design your wellness program?

Did you adopt the existing wellness program that your benefits provider included with their fees?

Did you consult with your employees to see what their wellness interests actually are? Are your employees getting well? How did you define "well?" How did you define "results?"

What criteria did you choose to measure?

The answers to these questions will help you see what the foundation of your wellness program is built on. Is it strong and stable? Was it built without much thought or input from future participants? Was it built on the premise of sustaining chronic illness with minimal symptoms or was it built on the foundation of reversing chronic illness and renewing the human body back to a state of wellness?

Yes, there is a big difference. The direction you choose will dictate not only your short term results for those seriously ill, it will also follow a predictable path of health or illness in those currently not seriously ill, both short and long term.

Let's take a closer look at how you defined "well" and "results" to see just how stable, secure, and long lasting your wellness foundation really is.

Well...What Do You Think?

Looking at perspectives on the concept of wellness shows us many different ideas of what it means to be well, get well, stay well, and to live well.

The only perspective that really matters in a company is the perspective of the top decision maker, usually the CEO.

Sounds harsh, yet, the reality is that where the CEO places high value is usually where the employees gravitate. When a CEO holds no value or no obvious use for something, such as his/her own health, employees will tend to shy away because of perceived lack of support, concern for job security, and even simply following the leader.

"Well" to one person may be a life free of disease and sickness. "Well" to another may be chronic illness controlled by medications to reduce symptoms, with colds and flu being the definition of "unwell."

How does the CEO of your company define "well?" That definition and the personal choices behind that definition reflect very good predictors of the effectiveness of that company's wellness program success.

Results and Returns

If a company wellness program defines "well" as chronic illness controlled by medications to reduce symptoms, with colds and flu being the definition of "unwell," what results and outcomes are you measuring for?

Do you consider effective results to be less cold and flu, or the presence of less symptoms of chronic illness that your employees still have?

Using medications to help alleviate symptoms of chronic illness is an ideal temporary measure, much like a cast on a broken bone. The cast allows for healing to happen and is removed after the bone has healed.

Drugs are not a long-term solution because they do not address the cause or the root of the chronic illness. They can effectively be used while lifestyle changes addressing the cause are introduced and implemented, with physician monitoring of drug reduction as healthy lifestyle results take effect.

Bumps in the Road

A picture is worth a thousand words, yet sometimes a single snapshot doesn't reveal the whole truth. Different people interpret pictures and words differently, not always as the artist or writer intended.

Here's a picture for you to consider. Have you ever driven on a highway covered by five to six inches of slush during the day? You can see tire tracks running all over the road, and now it is getting dark and the slush has almost frozen? Your car gets pulled in different directions no matter how hard you try steering in a straight line. No matter how focused, how careful, and how straight you drive, your car will follow the ruts on the road. Those ruts will still be there until they thaw or are cleared away.

Most everyone is familiar with driving through minor weather mishaps here and there, just as many of us are familiar with occasional minor health mishaps. Most of us, most of the time, drive on dry and clear roads. Similarly, most people don't feel the effects of chronic illness because they develop gradually and our bodies get acclimated to the way we feel.

We live our lives where we are comfortable with free and clear pathways wherever possible. It takes real effort and concentrated focus to stay the course while working to go a different direction, like creating healthy lifestyle changes.

Our neural pathways that have been made and worn deeply through years of repetitive behavior cannot be erased overnight – nor in reality can they be erased. New neural pathways must be provided and worked to become the current and more preferred pathways.

This is a simplistic explanation of behavior change that uses a basis in science with a heavy dose of common sense. Doing something new can be difficult and can seem like driving through an ice storm. The only thing worse would be if you were told to do it but didn't truly understand why, and you had to go it alone. Would you?

Why is Exercise an Afterthought?

The sum total of the need for regular exercise and the results of regular exercise are as relevant to the business as a whole as for the human body.

When one part of your business weakens or falls by the wayside, other parts of your business have to pick up the slack and get stressed by working overtime doing a job they weren't meant to do.

When one part of the human body process weakens or falls by the wayside, other parts of the human body have to pick up the slack and get stressed by working overtime doing a job they weren't meant to do.

Now that you have an idea of how you define "well," what results you are looking for, and the methods of dealing with chronic illness, let's stack that all up with another picture: why people don't exercise.

The Scandinavian Journal of Medicine & Science in Sports has published some interesting research that I urge you to read. Here is a small bit about what you will discover:

Evidence For Prescribing Exercise As Therapy In Chronic Disease. - Pedersen BK, Saltin B.

The Centre of Inflammation and Metabolism, Department of Infectious Diseases, Copenhagen, Denmark. bkp@rh.dk Comment in: Scand J Med Sci Sports. 2006 Jun;16(3):145-6.

Abstract

Considerable knowledge has accumulated in recent decades concerning the significance of physical activity in the treatment of a number of diseases, including diseases that do not primarily manifest as disorders of the locomotive apparatus. **In this review we present the evidence for prescribing exercise therapy in the treatment of metabolic syndrome-related disorders (insulin resistance, type 2 diabetes, dyslipidemia, hypertension, obesity), heart and pulmonary diseases (chronic obstructive pulmonary disease, coronary heart disease, chronic heart failure, intermittent claudication), muscle, bone and joint diseases (osteoarthritis, rheumatoid arthritis, osteoporosis, fibromyalgia, chronic fatigue syndrome) and cancer, depression, asthma and type 1 diabetes.** For each disease, we review the effect of exercise therapy on disease pathogenesis, on symptoms specific to the diagnosis, on physical fitness or strength and on quality of life. The possible mechanisms of action are briefly examined and the principles for prescribing exercise therapy are discussed, focusing on the type and amount of exercise and possible contraindications.

Visit   http://www.ncbi.nlm.nih.gov/pubmed/16451303   to view the entire 61 pages of research material.

The Importance and Value of a Fitness Trainer

Would your employees be able to do their jobs without ongoing training? Would they be able to produce quality work without education? If you didn't have to train them, does that mean they had previous training?

Even though we have all lived with our bodies since the beginning of our lives, most people know very little about how their body works, what it needs to stay healthy, what exercise actually is, or how to exercise.

Many people rely on "experts" like doctors who are scrambling to eke out five minutes maximum per patient and order appropriate tests in the order prescribed and allowed by insurance companies.

Often, people rely on television commercials to help them select the best medications for their particular "problems," seeing medications as a "quick fix" so they don't have to think about it anymore.

Only 30% of our population actually eats the daily amount of vegetables their body needs, and gets the amount of exercise their body needs for optimum health. Those are the people least likely to succumb to the top five causes of death, the least likely to cause increases in the insurance pools, and consequently, the least likely to be included in research studies. There is no profit to be made from someone who is well, when your business caters to the "unwell."

A qualified **Fitness Trainer** is able to help both fit and unfit employees exercise at their current fitness levels safely, while progressing them systematically to higher levels of fitness.

By using the services of a **Fitness Trainer**, your company can provide:

- A safe, customized plan for employees to follow

- Professional, individualized solutions

- Create an environment conducive to autonomy (motivation from within)

- Vitalized management and peer support

- Progress toward true wellness and well-being

Summary

Here's What We Know...

Regular Exercise and Proper Nutrition Decreases and/or Eliminates...

- Stress
- Risk of Heart Attack & Stroke
- Depression
- Hypertension (High Blood Pressure)
- Risk of Osteoporosis
- Joint Discomfort
- Risk of Breast Cancer by 60%
- Back Problems

Exercise Does More Than Simply Burn Calories!

Exercise Increases and Enhances...

- Mental Focus and Clarity
- Strength, Stamina & Energy
- Agility & Muscle Tone / Firmness
- Flexibility & Range of Motion
- Metabolic Rate
- Quality of Sleep
- Self Esteem and Confidence
- Immune System

Recipe for On-Site Corporate Fitness Success

Ingredients:

- One CEO with a mind for wellness
- One Employee Wellness Interest Survey
- One empty conference room or empty space
- One fitness trainer with on-site experience

Deliver CEO wellness message of support and follow up with Employee Wellness Survey.

After analysis, organize class schedules based on days and times preferred by employees and company.

Mix trainer with participants during weekly high-energy classes.

Serve with a nutrition program and a hefty portion of recognition and support.

Feeds: the company bottom line, morale, health, and well-being of all participants.

ABOUT THE AUTHOR

Greg Justice is an international best-selling author, speaker, and fitness entrepreneur. He opened AYC Health & Fitness, Kansas City's original personal training center, in May 1986, and has personally trained more than 48,000 one-on-one sessions. Today, AYC specializes in corporate wellness and personal training.

He has been actively involved in the fitness industry for more than a quarter of a century as a club manager, owner, personal fitness trainer, and corporate wellness supervisor. Greg currently serves on the advisory board of two personal training schools. He mentors and instructs trainers worldwide through his coaching programs and Corporate Boot Camp System class.

Greg has written articles for many fitness publications and websites. He is a featured columnist for Corporate Wellness Magazine. His monthly column, "Treadmill Talk," is published in Personal Fitness Professional magazine. He is the author of four books including *Mind Your Own Fitness, A Mindful Approach To Exercise*, and *Treadside Manner, Confessions Of A Serial Personal Trainer*.

Greg holds a master's degree in HPER (exercise science) and a bachelor's degree in Health & Physical Education from Morehead State University, Morehead, KY.